MW00414523

ENDOR.

Remedy: Freedom Through Deliverance

With the edge of experience, *Remedy* is not merely another good book on spiritual warfare. It contains tested wisdom needed to overcome your strong enemy. Beware: The contents inside are lethal and dangerous to the powers of darkness. **—James Goll, cofounder of Encounters Network and author of** *The Seer*, *Praying for Israel's Destiny*, **and** *Elijah's Revolution*

Remedy will help everyone who reads it come to a better understanding of the sovereign power of our God, His absolute authority, and the spiritual weapons He has given us. **—John Paul Jackson, founder of Streams Ministries International and host of** *Dreams and Mysteries*

Remedy weaves together biblical truths with the pragmatic to get Kingdom results. From the very beginning, it takes us on a journey on how to set those captives free. *Remedy* brings languages and understanding to Jesus' statement, "He who the Son sets free is free indeed." A must-read for every believer. **—Aaron Evans, founder, The Emerging Daniel Company**

I consider *Remedy* to be a significant tool to prepare the people of God to advance in victory. It is enlightening as well as equipping. With a rich history in spiritual deliverance, Michael and Bill French have put together an awesome tool to help anyone who is serious about advancing the Kingdom of God. This book is a refreshing combination of revelatory insights and scripture-based information, equipping the body of Christ to stand firm in the victory provided by Christ Jesus. This is a timely and significant book. I wholeheartedly recommend and not only reading, but also the implementation of these guidelines for victory. —**Bobby Conner, founder, Eagle's View Ministries**

It was with much anticipation that I looked forward to reading *Remedy*. Michael and Bill French bring much hands-on experience as well as biblical insight with understanding into the realm of the Spirit. There is a present call extended to the church to "come up here" to glean revelation and maturity essential for the end-time army of God. This book provides both. I highly recommend it for those who desire the high calling of God and fruitfulness in His Kingdom. —**Paul Keith Davis, founder, WhiteDove Ministries**

This book is a balanced, biblical, and long overdue treatment of a subject that has a history of abuse. The authors have carefully redressed the issue of spiritual warfare in a manner that will bless all who read it. *Remedy* and John Paul Jackson's *Needless Casualties of War* go hand-in-hand and will encourage those who have been confused in the area of deliverance. It is an excellent introduction to the subject and will particularly bless those who have struggled with fear of the devil rather than confidence in God. —**R.T. Kendall, former senior minister, Westminster Chapel, London, England**

Remedy:
Freedom Through Deliverance

Michael and Bill French
Copyright @ 2012 ShadeTree Publishing, LLC
Print ISBN: 978-1-937331-61-0
e-Book ISBN: 978-1-937331-62-7
Foreword by John Paul Jackson

Throughout this book, brackets [ ] represent the author's addition and are not part of the quoted scripture.

Scripture quotations marked KJV are taken from the Holy Bible, King James Version, 1768 edition, which is in the public domain.

Scripture quotations marked NKJV are taken from the Holy Bible, New King James Version, copyright © 1982 by Thomas Nelson, Inc. All rights reserved. Used by permission.

The purpose of this book is to educate and enlighten. This book is sold with the understanding that the author and publisher are not engaged in rendering counseling, albeit it professional or lay, to the reader or anyone else. The author and publisher shall have neither liability nor responsibility to any person or entity with respect to any loss or damage caused, or alleged to have been caused, directly or indirectly, by the information contained in this book.

Visit our Web site at www.ShadeTreePublishing.com.

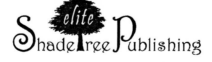

We dedicate this book to our wives, Joyce and Elisa, for their patience and commitment to us, without which we would never have been able to learn the principles contained in these pages.

Remedy: Freedom Through Deliverance

Foreword by John Paul Jackson 1

SECTION ONE KNOWING OUR ENEMY AND ALLIES 3

Chapter 1 WHO IS OUR ENEMY? 5

Chapter 2 DEMONS AND THE THINGS THEY DO 15

Chapter 3 WHO CAN BE AFFECTED BY THE
DEMONIC? 25

Chapter 4 WHO ARE OUR ALLIES? 33

SECTION TWO THE REMEDY 39

Chapter 5 CONFESSION, REPENTANCE, AND
FORGIVENESS 41

Chapter 6 SPIRITUAL AUTHORITY, POWER, AND
WEAPONS 49

**SECTION THREE PRACTICAL SUGGESTIONS ON
DELIVERANCE** 71

Chapter 7 ENGAGING IN MINISTRY 73

Chapter 8 HOW TO STAY FREE 83

Chapter 9 LIMITATIONS IN MINISTRY 91

Chapter 10 PUTTING IT ALL TO USE: PRACTICAL
ADVICE FROM A LIFETIME OF EXPERIENCE 107

FINAL THOUGHTS: WHAT DO I DO NOW? 125

About the Authors 129

Authors' Acknowledgments 129

References and Scriptures 133

Remedy: Freedom Through Deliverance

Foreword
by John Paul Jackson

"Behold, I give you the authority to trample on serpents and scorpions, and over all the power of the enemy, and nothing shall by any means hurt you."

—*Luke 10:19* NKJV

A believer's view of the demonic realm often falls into one of three categories: One type sees a demon in every shadow and ardently rebukes every cold draft. On the other end of the spectrum, another type has adopted a "Christian cavalier" mind-set and doesn't believe we can be attacked or even influenced by demons at all. Members of the third group are afraid to even mention Satan's name, just in case he's listening and comes after them with a pitchfork. Fortunately, none of these perspectives is accurate.

We are in a spiritual war. We fight this war every single day. Each one of us is involved in a moment-by-moment battle against an enemy that, for the most part, we don't see. We may feel him. We may even smell him. But we don't usually see him. His tactics are secretive, for that's how he works successfully. Once he has been exposed, he can be dealt with. And that is the truth Satan desperately tries to hide: God has given us authority over his power. Jesus didn't say, "I give you authority to tiptoe over all the power of the enemy" (which would have been sufficient), or, "I give you authority to walk over all the power of the enemy." No, instead Jesus declared, "I give you authority to trample all the power of the enemy."

We serve a God who has more authority and power over the demonic realm than we could ever humanly imagine. Comparing His power to any other would be like comparing a B-2 stealth bomber to a child's paper airplane. Demons tremble at the mere mention of His name. However, for millennia, Satan has skillfully managed to overexert, blind, and scare many believers. We have experienced more than a little confusion over our God-given authority. Jesus never intended His bride to be wrapped up in, ignorant of, or scared of the demonic realm. Instead, He gave us authority to stand up to the devil's schemes and reveal his lies for what they truly are.

God's power and authority over the demonic realm are wonderfully displayed and fantastically obvious in the Gospels. One of Jesus' most prolific ministries on earth was that of deliverance, setting the captives free. The demon-possessed would see Him from far off, throw themselves at His feet, and try to distract or delay their departure by physically manifesting in their hosts. But Jesus was not distracted; the enemy was still cast out.

Imagine walking with God to the extent that when the enemy sees the power of God in you, he panics and falls on his face. This is the authority Jesus wielded—the authority He granted us so we could trample the enemy's power. *Remedy: Freedom Through Deliverance*, by my good friends Michael and Bill French, will help everyone who reads it come to a better understanding of the sovereign power of our God, His absolute authority, and the spiritual weapons He has given us to turn back the battle at the gate.

About John Paul Jackson
John Paul Jackson is a husband, father, and established authority on Christian spirituality and dream interpretation. His biblical approach to dreams reveals their life-changing purpose, and restores an overlooked way God chooses to communicate with people. John Paul's teachings have stirred and renewed passion for God among people of all ages from various faith backgrounds. His thoughtful "explanations of the unexplainable" and simple, yet profound concepts help people relate to God and each other in fresh ways. As an author, speaker, and television guest, John Paul has impacted hundreds of thousands of people, emphasizing character as a key element in the true spiritual life. His many years of study and experience have made him a respected and sought-after spiritual advisor to leaders and believers around the world. John Paul has shared his practical and spiritual expertise with an international audience through the Streams Training Center courses and publications. For more information about John Paul, visit www.streamsministries.com.

SECTION ONE
KNOWING OUR ENEMY AND ALLIES

Deliverance ministry is a touchy subject for most of the Church world. Just mention the word *deliverance*, and many people conjure up images of *The Exorcist* and other media stereotypes. The confusion, fear, and anxiety caused by these associations are a tactic of the enemy to keep people from understanding the depths of God's power. Deliverance doesn't need to be a scary subject—it just needs to be better understood. We need to replace the mythology surrounding deliverance with the reality of God's Word.

Section One of this book deals with the foundational biblical elements of deliverance ministry. It will answer questions such as:

- Are the devil and demons real?
- If so, what do they do?
- What impact does this have on me as a Christian?

In order to understand deliverance ministry and its place in the contemporary Church, we need to begin with a biblical definition and show why deliverance is a valid and necessary ministry.

CHAPTER 1
WHO IS OUR ENEMY?

Over the years, many people have argued that it is inappropriate to discuss the topic of knowing our enemy. They feel that time spent discussing the devil glorifies him instead of God, but it is important to remember that only the untrained soldier does not seek to understand his or her adversary.

God's Word repeatedly compares the believer with a soldier actively engaged in warfare.[1] It is important to know that one aspect of being a competent soldier in God's army requires recognizing the nature of the enemy and his tactics, as well as what motivates him to steal, kill, and destroy.[2]

The Attributes of Satan

God's Word provides a limited amount of information regarding Satan's origin. Isaiah 14 and Ezekiel 28 present the idea that Satan, once known as Lucifer, existed before the events of Genesis 1. At the time of the writing of Isaiah and Ezekiel, Jewish authors used a device called parallel semantics, which enabled two histories to be narrated as one. For example, Isaiah 14 tells the story of the Babylonian kingdom, an ancient kingdom that was evil and corrupt. But these verses also describe the fall of Lucifer and how he became Satan. In Ezekiel 28, we find the story of the kingdom of Tyre, an equally evil and corrupt nation. Here, too, is the story of Lucifer's fall. Both chapters describe two subjects (Lucifer and the kingdoms) in one writing.

Based on Isaiah 14 and Ezekiel 28, it appears that Lucifer was a powerful angel (on a similar level as the archangel Michael) who sought to exalt himself to the level of God, but instead, he fell from heaven.

If Gabriel is identified as the great messenger angel and Michael as the great warrior angel, then Lucifer would be identified as the great worship angel.

> *...The workmanship of your timbrels and pipes was prepared for you on the day you were created...*
> —*Ezekiel 28:13* NKJV

This verse associates Lucifer with music and worship. When we examine Satan's activities on the earth today, we recognize that one of his primary tools is music and its influence on humankind. Scripture also indicates that Lucifer was a beautiful being and his beauty was one of the causes of his downfall.

> *Every precious stone was your covering: The sardius, topaz, and diamond, beryl, onyx, and jasper, sapphire, turquoise, and emerald with*

gold... Your heart was lifted up because of your beauty; you corrupted your wisdom for the sake of your splendor
—*Ezekiel 28:13, 17* NKJV

Lucifer was a powerful being "who made the earth tremble, who shook kingdoms, who made the world as a wilderness and destroyed its cities."[3]

Lucifer boasts that he will exalt his throne above the stars of God.

For you have said in your heart: "I will ascend into heaven, I will exalt my throne above the stars of God; I will also sit on the mount of the congregation on the farthest sides of the north; I will ascend above the heights of the clouds, I will be like the Most High."
—*Isaiah 14:13–14* NKJV

What does a throne symbolize? Authority and dominion. It is this attitude of pride (notice the phrase *I will* appears five times in these two verses) that results in Lucifer's downfall. He believed he could be "like the Most High," that he could be equal with God.

Satan was also persuasive. He convinced one-third of the host of heaven that he could be equal with God. He lured them to follow him in rebellion and, ultimately, to be cast out with him.[4]

Satan's Primary Role in the Earth

Isaiah 14 and Ezekiel 28 describe who Satan was before the fall. However, this book focuses more on what he is doing in the present. Romans 11:29 teaches us that "the gifts and the calling of God are irrevocable" (NKJV). According to this scriptural principle, Satan may very well retain much of the power, authority, and persuasiveness he was given as Lucifer, a highly attractive being.

God's Word also refers to "all the power of the enemy"[5] and Satan transforming himself "into an angel of light.[6] If Satan maintains at least some of the power, authority, and persuasiveness he operated in prior to the fall, believers must be prepared for the deployment of those skills today.

Zechariah 3 offers the first clue to how Satan's purposes operate in the earth. Consider the cleansing of Joshua, the high priest.

> *Then he showed me Joshua the high priest standing before the Angel of the LORD, and Satan standing at his right hand to oppose him.*
> —*Zechariah 3:1 NKJV*

It is unlikely that any of us individually is important enough for Satan to come in person to oppose us. Yet, opposition to God's servants is a huge priority of Satan and his minions.

Satan is not omnipotent, omniscient, or omnipresent as are God the Father, Son, and Holy Spirit. However, since one-third of the heavenly host fell with him, he does have sufficient help all over the globe and in the heavens to oppress God's servants.

When we, as believers, decide to walk more closely with the Lord in loving obedience and to faithfully act in conjunction with God's call on our lives, we can reasonably assume Satan (or more likely, one of his representatives) will attack us. So, it becomes extremely important for us not only to know our enemy, but to know ourselves and the authority in which God has designed us to walk. The believer's authority will be discussed more fully in Chapter 6.

Satan's Primary Tool

Satan, the adversary, made his first appearance to Adam and Eve in Genesis 3. He came in the form of a serpent with language ability (something that must not have been highly unusual since Eve seemed quite comfortable with his presence). He was probably standing upright, since he was shortly thereafter condemned to crawl on his belly for the rest of his life. Adam and Eve were still walking in innocence and clothed in nothing more than the glory of the Lord. However, something was about to happen that would forever strip them of their innocence and reveal their nakedness.

This is the story of Adam's loss of his kingdom to the devious and persuasive serpent, Satan. We see that Satan's powers of persuasion were cloaked in innuendo, half-truths, and lies. He still consistently uses these tactics to oppose God's servants. He weaves these lies well and seeks to subtly cast doubt upon God's Word.

> *Now the serpent was more cunning than any beast of the field which the LORD God had made. And he said to the woman, "Has God indeed said, 'You shall not eat of every tree of the garden'?" And the woman said to the serpent, "We may eat the fruit of the trees of the garden; but of the fruit of the tree which is in the midst of the garden, God has said, 'You shall not eat it, nor shall you touch it, lest you die.'" Then the serpent said to the woman, "You will not surely die. For God knows that in the day you eat of it your eyes will be opened, and you will be like God, knowing good and evil."*
>
> *—Genesis 3:1–5 NKJV*

In Satan's first deception, he asked, "Is it really true? Has God *really* said you cannot eat from every tree in the garden?" Already confused, Eve responded that she may not eat of it, nor touch it. This was not what God had said to Adam and Eve,[7] but now Satan had a base from which to work. He immediately began to question God's meaning: "Does God really care about you? If He did, wouldn't He let you eat from all the trees? Do you really believe you would die if you ate from this tree?" This mind-set of selfish ambition cast doubt and suspicion on God's Word, which is the primary tool the enemy uses to oppose those who choose to serve Almighty God.

Satan's final ploy was a direct attack on God's Word: "You will not surely die." Yet spiritual death came immediately, and physical death became the common experience of humanity. While some still question the accuracy of the account because Adam's physical death did not occur on that literal day, the Bible states, "With the Lord one day is as a thousand years."[8] From that time on, no person has ever lived beyond a thousand years. This verse also makes one other thing abundantly clear: God exists outside our understanding of time.

Can Satan Read Our Minds?

If Satan cannot oppose God's chosen ones through deception, then his next endeavor is to kill them. Genesis 3 explains why Satan seeks to destroy God's servants.

> *"And I will put enmity between you and the woman, and between your seed and her Seed; He shall bruise your head, and you shall bruise His heel."*
>
> —Genesis 3:15 NKJV

Satan's efforts to destroy the woman's Seed reveals another important piece of information about our adversary. Genesis 3:15 contains the first prophecy of the coming Messiah: The Seed of the woman "shall bruise your head, and you shall bruise His heel." To Satan, Cain and Abel appeared to be the Seed of the woman, so he provoked Cain to kill Abel. Satan was trying to kill the Seed, but he failed.

When Moses was born and the spirit world began to sense the excitement of a deliverer arriving upon the scene, Satan assumed Moses was the Seed. Satan entered the heart of Pharaoh and compelled him to seek to kill all the Hebrew male infants. Neither Satan's nor Pharaoh's plan succeeded.

Next, we see the true Messiah born in a manger in Bethlehem. Once again, Satan struck out against the children, and once again he was unsuccessful. Each time God prepared to bring forth a mighty work of deliverance, Satan sought to oppose it by killing the children. He used this strategy in an attempt to destroy the Seed—the Deliverer, God's Servant—who would be the vessel to bring forth freedom.

Today, thousands of children are killed each year at the hands of abortionists. Does our adversary again feel that something is on the horizon in the spiritual world?

What we learn from this is clear: Satan cannot read your mind. If he could, he would not have failed in all the attempts to kill the Seed that God referred to in the garden. Unquestionably, certain people knew who and where the Messiah was. Mary and Joseph knew, and so did Elizabeth and the shepherds. Yet Satan failed as a result of imperfect knowledge. He could not read the minds of those who knew the Christ, and he cannot read the minds of men and women today. He has, however, had thousands of years to become an expert on human behavior. He will use this knowledge to attempt to persuade men and women that he knows exactly what they are thinking and give credibility to the subtle lies he uses so well.

Are There Limits to Satan's Authority?

Satan opposes God's servants primarily through deception; however, he is not all-powerful. There are limits to Satan's authority. We find an excellent reference in the book of Job that answers this question and also provides other insights about the areas from which Satan operates.

The first thing we learn is that Satan still has access to God's throne.

> *Now there was a day when the sons of God came to present themselves before the LORD, and Satan also came among them. And the LORD*

> *said to Satan, "From where do you come?" So Satan answered the LORD and said, "From going to and fro on the earth, and from walking back and forth on it."*
>
> —*Job 1:6–7 NKJV*

Satan has been roaming about the earth and has now come to present himself before the Lord. This Scripture provides significant information when we recognize that Satan operates both on earth and in heavenly realms, but more important is what comes next:

> *Then the LORD said to Satan, "Have you considered My servant Job, that there is none like him on the earth, a blameless and upright man, one who fears God and shuns evil?" So Satan answered the LORD and said, "Does Job fear God for nothing? Have You not made a hedge around him, around his household, and around all that he has on every side? You have blessed the work of his hands, and his possessions have increased in the land. But now, stretch out Your hand and touch all that he has, and he will surely curse You to Your face!" And the LORD said to Satan, "Behold, all that he has is in your power; only do not lay a hand on his person." So Satan went out from the presence of the LORD.*
>
> —*Job 1:8–12 NKJV*

Here we find clear proof that Satan's authority in connection with God's servants is limited.

Job 1 details an interesting exchange between God and Satan regarding Job. In that conversation, it is important to note that it was God, not Satan, who brought up the issue of Job. The Lord Himself pointed out His choice servant to the enemy. Satan reacted by asking permission to come against Job. This point is remarkable. Job was protected from the attacks of the enemy until Satan received permission to act, and even then his actions were limited: "only do not lay a hand on his person."

This isn't the only example of the Lord allowing the enemy to test His servants. Recall Peter's conversation with Jesus. The Lord said that Satan had asked permission to sift Peter as wheat.[9] That request apparently had been granted, since the Lord reminded Peter that He had prayed for him, that his faith would not fail during the sifting process.[10] Jesus further advised Peter that when he had returned to Him, he was to strengthen the believers. In effect, Jesus said, "Peter, I have allowed this! Satan can do what he will, but he can go only so far. Afterward, Peter, you will return to Me." It was after this that Peter, who denied Christ on multiple occasions, later became one of the pillars of the faith.

In the examples and circumstances of both Job and Peter, we find limitations on the authority Satan had in testing them. In both cases, Satan understood a line existed that he could not cross. Satan's authority to test and try was, and still is, limited. God had already set the limitations, and only He or Job could have extended them. Had Job complained in bitterness and rebellion, it would have extended the boundary of Satan's authority. Instead, Job endured and remained faithful. Having suffered what was sent against him, Job said, "Naked I came from my mother's womb, and naked shall I return there. The LORD gave, and the LORD has taken away; blessed be the name of the LORD."[11]

Satan, knowing his limitations, later returned to the Lord and asked for the line to be moved.[12] Even after God increased the limits, Job didn't sin with his lips. He was confronted by his friends and his wife, and could have easily moved the line by saying, "This is too much," but instead he stood firm. Job embodied the commandment of Ephesians 6:13 in that he stood, and having done all, continued to stand.

Christians should not become confused or despondent when Satan is granted limited authority to *sift* them, for God will use the event to purify and prepare His vessels for greater use. Satan is the devourer who has come to steal, kill, and destroy. If we are walking in rebellion, we grant him access to wreak havoc. Even if we are living in obedience, there are times in our lives when God allows him to assault us, saying, "You have My permission, but you cannot go beyond this point." In times of testing, when we want to blame Satan, it is wise to first ask God if He is allowing this process to teach us. Job lost much, but in the end, the Lord restored to him twice as much as he had before. Why? First, Job stood and, having done all, continued to stand; and second, he turned away from selfishness.

Isaiah 14 and Ezekiel 28 paint a graphic picture of the being who would later be known as Satan. The biblical portrait of Satan is one many people would prefer not to see. Instead of a strong, authoritative, destructive being with tremendous powers of persuasion, the world chooses to see a somewhat foolish imp dressed in a red suit and carrying a pitchfork. This image is exactly what our enemy would like God's army to see. Through it, he has convinced many that he is a fairy tale, dead or incompetent, and so he isn't perceived as a threat.

If we are to stand against the devil, we must expect him to oppose us at every turn and that his primary weapon will be deception.[13] While Satan is not omnipresent and cannot read our minds, he still has access to the heavenly realms. He uses that access and his cunning to direct his forces against God's saints. So, why is he here at all? Wouldn't it be much easier on us if Satan didn't exist? Consider this—how would we grow if we had no adversary? A kitchen knife is not sharpened on a stick of butter, but rather against an abrasive stone. And so it is with our lives.

CHAPTER 2

DEMONS AND THE THINGS THEY DO

Both the Old and New Testaments attest to the existence of demons. Two Hebrew words are translated "demon" or "devil": (1) *shed* (shade): a demon, malignant, devil[14]; and (2) *sair* (saw-eer'): shaggy, a he-goat, faun, devil, or satyr.[15] The primary Greek word translated "demon" or "devil" in the New Testament is *daimonion* (dahee-mon'-ee-on): a demonic being, a deity, devil, or god.[16] From these original language words as used in Scripture, it is clear that a demon is a spirit being that seeks to set itself up as a god in individuals' lives. Its true intention is to bring about destruction (notice that the Hebrew word *shed* can also be translated as "malignant").[17]

God's Word does not give the specific origin of demons. However, we can assume these beings are the third of the heavenly host that fell with Lucifer after he enticed them to follow him in his rebellion. We can also assume that Satan remains their leader. In fact, God's Word strongly suggests that demonic ranks are structured in military form with Satan as the head, chief, or general. Ephesians lays the foundation for this view.

> *For we do not wrestle against flesh and blood, but against principalities, against powers, against the rulers of the darkness of this age, against spiritual hosts of wickedness in the heavenly places.*
>
> —*Ephesians 6:12 NKJV*

Though Scripture does not paint a precise picture of the demonic realm, we can glean much about demons and their actions from various passages. From this study of the demonic realm, one theme becomes clear: Demons follow the direction of their master, the devil, and seek to do his bidding. Satan came "to steal, and kill, and destroy,"[18] and so these are the primary tasks of his minions, as well.

Do Demons Still Exist on the Earth Today?

Some people still wonder whether demons exist in the world, but the pervasiveness and openness of occult activity is a sufficient answer to that question. For those who seek scriptural proof, God's Word contains much evidence of the continued existence and activity of demons.

Until the prophecies of John in the book of Revelation are fulfilled, Satan and his demonic hordes remain loosed upon the earth. Revelation 20 describes the ultimate fate of Satan and his forces, and most biblical scholars agree that the events leading to Satan's captivity have not yet been fulfilled. So, both present-day physical evidence and biblical prophecy confirm that demons remain loosed upon the earth and are presently active. It also seems that while demons' activity may have taken on different manifestations, their goals and functions remain the same. The following scriptural examples support this view.

The reader can glean a great deal from Jesus' encounter with the two demon-possessed men in Matthew 8.

> *When He had come to the other side, to the country of the Gergesenes, there met Him two demon-possessed men, coming out of the tombs, exceedingly fierce, so that no one could pass that way. And suddenly they cried out, saying, "What have we to do with You, Jesus, You Son of God? Have You come here to torment us before the time?" Now a good way off from them there was a herd of many swine feeding. So the demons begged Him, saying, "If You cast us out, permit us to go away into the herd of swine." And He said to them, "Go." So when they had come out, they went into the herd of swine. And suddenly the whole herd of swine ran violently down the steep place into the sea, and perished in the water. Then those who kept them fled; and they went away into the city and told everything, including what had happened to the demon-possessed men. And behold, the whole city came out to meet Jesus. And when they saw Him, they begged Him to depart from their region.*
>
> *—Matthew 8:28–34 NKJV*

This account provides insight about what demons do. Verse 28 begins by identifying these men as being "exceedingly fierce," or violent. These violent tendencies resulted from the demonic pressure overwhelming the men. The passage then conveys that the men "cried out," or shouted (verse 29). This must have been demons speaking through them, since the men themselves were not being tormented by Jesus. The demons were able to detect two points of information that the people did not: (1) They recognized Jesus as the Son of God, and (2) there is an appointed time for their torment.

Verse 31 confirms that demons were acting through these men, since they petitioned Jesus about where they should be sent. Apparently, demons have something akin to emotions or feelings because they "begged" Jesus, pleading, "If You cast us out..." There was never any question about Jesus' ability to drive them out, so their statement was a tactic to delay. Certainly these demons knew they had to go whether they wanted to or not.

What might easily be overlooked in this account is where the demons were found, and then, where they were sent. When Jesus appeared on the scene, these demons were occupying the bodies of men. We then learn that demons can occupy or inhabit animal bodies, as well ("they went into the herd of swine"). Today these conclusions are still controversial just as they were in Jesus' time; this deliverance wrought such upheaval that "the whole city" came out and implored Jesus to vacate their region.

Examination of the passage in Matthew 8 indicates one thing for certain: demonic entities intend to destroy the lives of those they seek to control. In this case, the two men were driven to live apart from society in a very undesirable location (in the midst of the tombs). While this lifestyle was certainly not what these individuals would have chosen, they were manipulated and coerced into it. This same destructive goal is being pursued by demonic powers today.

An often-unwitting introduction to the demonic realm occurs by using occult objects such as an Ouija board. While often considered merely a game, this board accesses an immersion into the occult that is far from innocent, no matter the context of its use. The following example shows how dabbling in "innocent" occult games can produce life-altering consequences and illustrates how demons are at work even today.

Bill was asked by a psychiatrist who worked with his ministry to meet with a young woman seeking release from a psychiatric hospital. The woman explained that she did not desire to be in the psychiatric ward and added that her problems had originated from playing with an Ouija board. She quickly realized that the board was actually answering her questions, and ultimately, the demonic entity controlling the board advised her that if she played a certain form of rock music, the board would become more effective. She did, and it did. Next, the board said that if she would place some of her blood on it, it would become even more effective. Once again she did, and it did. In the end, her arms were covered with scars from this induced bloodletting, and she became a resident at an "undesirable" location, all through demonic manipulation. Sounds like a modern-day Matthew 8.

Sickness, Disease, and Death

The narrative in Matthew 9 provides additional information about what demons do.

> As they went out, behold, they brought to Him a man, mute and demon-possessed. And when the demon was cast out, the mute spoke. And the multitudes marveled, saying, "It was never seen like this in Israel!" But the Pharisees said, "He casts out demons by the ruler of the demons."
>
> —Matthew 9:32–34 NKJV

In these verses, we learn that demons can render an individual sick. Notice Jesus did not say, "Be healed," but the verse records that "after the demon was cast out, the mute could speak."

Now, let's look at the account of the woman with the spirit of disease.

> And behold, there was a woman who had a spirit of infirmity eighteen years, and was bent over and could in no way raise herself up. But when Jesus saw her, He called her to Him and said to her, "Woman, you are loosed from your

> *infirmity." And He laid His hands on her, and immediately she was made straight, and glorified God.*
>
> —*Luke 13:11–13* NKJV

Taken together, these verses show that demons have the power to cause sickness and disease. While we cannot infer that every illness is brought on by some demonic oppression, these passages demonstrate that inducing physical infirmities is one of the weapons demons use to destroy an individual. A number of other scriptures confirm this demonic function (i.e., Matthew 12:22 and Matthew 17:14–18).

Mark's Gospel provides additional insight into the demonic world's ultimate goal. The following passage recounts the story of the epileptic boy who was brought to Jesus by his father.

> *Then one of the crowd answered and said, "Teacher, I brought You my son, who has a mute spirit. And wherever it seizes him, it throws him down; he foams at the mouth, gnashes his teeth, and becomes rigid. So I spoke to Your disciples, that they should cast it out, but they could not." He answered him and said, "O faithless generation, how long shall I be with you? How long shall I bear with you? Bring him to Me." Then they brought him to Him. And when he saw Him, immediately the spirit convulsed him, and he fell on the ground and wallowed, foaming at the mouth. So He asked his father, "How long has this been happening to him?" And he said, "From childhood. And often he has thrown him both into the fire and into the water to destroy him. But if You can do anything, have compassion on us and help us." Jesus said to him, "If you can believe, all things are possible to him who believes." Immediately the father of the child cried out and said with tears, "Lord, I*

*believe; help my unbelief!" When Jesus saw that
the people came running together, He rebuked
the unclean spirit, saying to it, "Deaf and dumb
spirit, I command you, come out of him and enter
him no more!" Then the spirit cried out,
convulsed him greatly, and came out of him. And
he became as one dead, so that many said, "He
is dead." But Jesus took him by the hand and
lifted him up, and he arose.*

—*Mark 9:17–27* NKJV

Here we find the demonic presence causing seizures, but
more interesting still is the action taken by this demon as
Jesus commanded it to come out: the spirit cried out, and
as it left the child, it made him appear dead. As we have
seen, Satan's primary weapon is deception. In this case,
either as a final act of demonic falsehood or as a result of
the previous manifestation, the boy seemed to have died,
giving the appearance of demonic victory. But, Jesus saw
through this guise and lifted the boy up. There is no
scriptural evidence to verify that demons by themselves can
cause a person's death, yet this simple deception indicates
that it is most certainly their goal, and they might have
succeeded in this case if God's power hadn't intervened.

Demonic Activities on the Earth Today

We must remember that demons act in accordance with
their evil nature, the purpose of which is theft, death, and
destruction. They will operate in any way that furthers
these goals. The Bible is the most important source of
information regarding a demon's actions. However, many
of the manifestations described in the Word have been seen
in the course of modern-day ministry. Current ministry
examples convince us that the demonic world is still alive
and well and also provide insight into other areas where
the demonic is active, even if those areas are not explicitly
stated in Scripture.

On one occasion, Bill met with a young man who was under the influence of a demonic entity that caused him to act like a werewolf. The young man would actually go outside at night and howl at the moon, and the hair on his body began to grow extraordinarily long. He also displayed unusual knowledge of the tragic event when several Russian cosmonauts died in space. This young man described in intricate detail exactly what had caused their death and the condition of their bodies—before they had been recovered. When the bodies were recovered, the young man's information proved accurate. When asked how he had known, the young man replied, "I went out there." This story indicates that demons assist individuals in the practice known as astral projection.

Another occasion highlighted demonic supernatural strength. During this encounter, Bill, who was six feet tall and weighed approximately two hundred fifty pounds at the time, was ministering to a woman who was five feet two and weighed about one hundred thirty pounds. Both were sitting in folding chairs directly across from each other. While Bill was praying for her, the woman slid her foot under the metal bar between the front legs of Bill's folding chair, and with a flip of her foot, sent Bill suddenly flying across the room and into the wall. This action was performed with enough force that the plastic feet from the end of the folding chair legs remained on the floor. Obviously, this display of supernatural strength was intended to harm Bill, but he remained completely uninjured.

The phenomenon of feigned death has been observed in present-day ministry situations, as well. One evening when our team was ministering to a young man who complained of an inability to worship, he fell from his chair and lay on the floor for an hour. Nothing the ministry team said or did had any impact. A few weeks later, the young man returned for ministry, and when Bill began to minister to him, he again fell to the floor. A police officer assisting with the ministry immediately shouted out, "It's a spirit of death!" When the officer proclaimed what the Lord had revealed to him, the young man began to take on very real symptoms of death. His body became rigid; all signs of breathing ceased, and it appeared that the blood in his limbs had begun to settle. Although this was disturbing, the team stood on the authority of God's Word and continued to minister. Ultimately, the young man was loosed from this spirit of death and received freedom from demonic oppression. He later became a worship leader in a local church. This example doesn't prove whether or not a demon can actually cause death, but it does make clear that they can certainly impose the appearance of death.

The following summary provides a partial list of things demons do, as identified by God's Word:

- They speak (Matthew 8:29).
- They lie (John 8:44).
- They argue or question (Matthew 8:29–31).
- They have supernatural strength (Mark 5:3).
- They cause violence (Matthew 8:28).
- They cause sickness and disease (Luke 13:11; Mark 9:20).
- They control bodily functions (Mark 9:20–22).
- They have recognition (Matthew 8:29).
- They know their end (Matthew 8:29).
- They may possess things or creatures other than humans (Matthew 8:32).
- They intend to cause death and destruction (Matthew 8:32).
- They cause self-mutilation (Mark 5:5).
- They have names (Mark 5:9).
- They cause muteness and blindness (Matthew 12:22).
- They cause foaming at the mouth (Mark 9:18).
- They cause the appearance of death (Mark 9:26).

Remedy: Freedom Through Deliverance

This list is important in helping us understand that demons act and function as intelligent beings. If we as believers are going to perform the wonders Jesus did, we must be prepared to see the spiritual activities He saw.

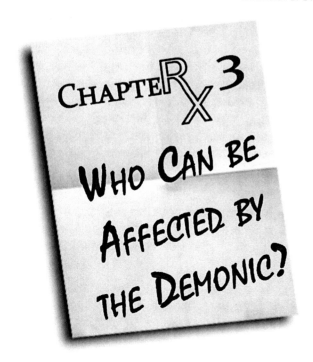

CHAPTER 3

WHO CAN BE AFFECTED BY THE DEMONIC?

Since the primary purpose of the demonic world is to steal, kill, and destroy, the next logical question is, "Who is the primary target of its attack?" Over the years, discussion about demons has raged in the Christian community, but no definitive answer has been reached as to who can be affected or afflicted by them, especially since their hostile takeovers are frequently denoted by the word *possessed*. Before we discuss how a demon can influence an individual and what makes an individual susceptible to that influence, let's examine the scriptural basis for *possession* and *oppression*.

Possessed versus Oppressed

The English word *possessed* implies absolute ownership or control (in this case, of the spirit, soul, and flesh), so it is difficult to believe a Christian could be possessed by a demon. At the same time, evidence abounds, much of it confirmed by Scripture, that Christians can be demonically influenced. Every time the Greek word *daimonizomai* (dahee-mon-id'-zom-ahee), translated "possessed," occurs in the New Testament, it refers to the demonic realm (with two notable exceptions—Acts 8:7 and 16:16—where *echo* is used, meaning "to hold"). Although *daimonizomai* is usually translated as "possessed," the actual definition is "to be exercised by a demon—have a (be vexed with, be possessed with) devil(s)." It can also indicate being demonized, annoyed, troubled, or tormented.[19]

Christians, by definition, are owned by Jesus Christ; in other words, they may be disturbed, harassed, and certainly annoyed or plagued by demonic influence, but not owned or possessed.

For clarity, this book will use the terms *possessed* and *oppressed* to delineate the influence a demon can have over an individual. While *possession* implies total, absolute control by the possessor, *oppression* implies harassment, intimidation, and manipulation. Unfortunately, believers can succumb to oppression to such a degree that it can be difficult to distinguish between the two.

Can Nonbelievers Have Demons?

The answer is yes. If individuals haven't accepted Jesus' redemption, they are subject to the ruler of this world; therefore, nonbelievers clearly can be oppressed or possessed by demons. Several scriptures prove this; Mark 7:24–30 is the most clear:

> *From there He arose and went to the region of Tyre and Sidon. And He entered a house and wanted no one to know it, but He could not be hidden. For a woman whose young daughter had an unclean spirit heard about Him, and she came and fell at His feet. The woman was a Greek, a Syro-Phoenician by birth, and she kept asking Him to cast the demon out of her*

daughter. But Jesus said to her, "Let the children be filled first, for it is not good to take the children's bread and throw it to the little dogs." And she answered and said to Him, "Yes, Lord, yet even the little dogs under the table eat from the children's crumbs." Then He said to her, "For this saying go your way; the demon has gone out of your daughter." And when she had come to her house, she found the demon gone out, and her daughter lying on the bed.
—Mark 7:24–30 NKJV

This woman was Greek, a Syro-Phoenician Gentile. Her daughter had a demon (an unclean spirit), of which she was beseeching Jesus to "cast out." Since neither she nor her daughter was a covenant-keeping Jew, Jesus tells her that the deliverance she requests is the "children's bread." Yet, because she put her faith in Him, the child was set free.[20] This passage establishes two significant points: (1) nonbelievers can have demons, and (2) Jesus has authority even in the life of the nonbeliever.

This passage also suggests that nonbelievers typically are not the ones to whom deliverance is offered. In this context, we see that even though Jesus' role was to minister first to the Jewish people, He will also extend His touch to all humankind. However, deliverance is not the first step—acknowledging our faith in Christ is. The woman's statement indicates that she placed her trust in Jesus, that He was sufficient even for her, and only after her declaration of faith was Jesus willing to grant her request. As will be developed in a later chapter, it is very important for the one receiving ministry to believe in Jesus and His authority. Otherwise, casting out demons can potentially do more harm than good.

Can Christians Be Controlled by Demons?

Ephesians 4:30 clearly shows that when someone's life has been turned over to Christ, that person has been sealed for the day of redemption. But it is important that we understand just what part of us has been sealed.

> *Now He who establishes us with you in Christ and has anointed us is God, who also has sealed us and given us the Spirit in our hearts as a guarantee.*
> —*2 Corinthians 1:21–22* NKJV

As this verse indicates, the heart (or spirit) of a person is sealed for the day of redemption and is the dwelling place of the Holy Spirit. The Holy Spirit and a demonic spirit cannot occupy the same space. However, the Holy Spirit inhabits only the heart (or spirit) of a believer and not the mind or flesh. Paul wrote that our whole being needs to be sanctified.

> *Now may the God of peace Himself sanctify you completely; and may your whole spirit, soul, and body be preserved blameless at the coming of our Lord Jesus Christ.*
> —*1 Thessalonians 5:23* NKJV

Nowhere does Scripture indicate that our mind and flesh are sealed like our spirit. In fact, it is just the opposite (see Romans 7:15–25). So, these two areas—the mind and flesh—are battlegrounds, and warfare is continually conducted to determine who (or what) will rule: either the divine will of God or the human will of the soul. As long as we continue to submit our mind and flesh to the Holy Spirit's rule, they are outside demonic jurisdiction; nonetheless, as contested ground, they may be minefields in which our adversary can operate.

We must be careful to keep our mind and flesh directed in the ways of the Lord and to focus steadfastly on Him. Paul counsels that nothing good dwells in our flesh[21] and that we should not allow the flesh to fulfill its lusts.[22] Left to its own devices, the flesh is not subject to the Holy Spirit, and we must align it with the Spirit's will daily.

Since Paul also admonished us not to be conformed to this world but to be transformed by the renewing of our minds[23] and that the carnal mind is at enmity with God,[24] evidently putting on the mind of Christ is a battle.[25] If we do not maintain the freshness of this divine relationship through communion in prayer and Scripture, the enemy may temporarily, and in a limited fashion, take "possession" of our flesh or mind. However, he cannot do so without us knowingly or unknowingly giving consent. Cognizant consent entails willful rebellion and sin, and choosing to walk under the control of our soul rather than the Spirit's leading. Unknowing consent means failing to disallow our fleshly lusts or to not conscientiously pursue the renewing of our mind, even though we are not purposefully meaning to rebel.

We can conclude, then, that Christians can have anything they choose or consent (knowingly or unknowingly) to have; consequently, Christians can have demons. It is biblically sound to say that believers can be oppressed, tormented, or hindered, but not totally possessed by demons; however, depending on how much authority and control they have relinquished to the enemy, believers may appear to be possessed. For example, let's again examine the story of the woman in Luke 13.

> *And behold, there was a woman who had a spirit of infirmity eighteen years, and was bent over and could in no way raise herself up. But when Jesus saw her, He called her to Him and said to her, "Woman, you are loosed from your infirmity." And He laid His hands on her, and immediately she was made straight, and glorified God. But the ruler of the synagogue answered with indignation, because Jesus had healed on the Sabbath; and he said to the crowd, "There are six days on which men ought to work; therefore come and be healed on them, and not on the Sabbath day." The Lord then*

> *answered him and said, "Hypocrite! Does not each one of you on the Sabbath loose his ox or donkey from the stall, and lead it away to water it? So ought not this woman, being a daughter of Abraham, whom Satan has bound—think of it— for eighteen years, be loosed from this bond on the Sabbath?" And when He said these things, all His adversaries were put to shame; and all the multitude rejoiced for all the glorious things that were done by Him.*
>
> *—Luke 13:11–17* NKJV

The apostle Paul states, "Therefore know that only those who are of faith are sons of Abraham";[26] that is to say, if you are a believer as Abraham was, you are a son or daughter of Abraham. Therefore, the woman mentioned in Luke 13 must be a person of faith because she is called by Jesus Himself a "daughter of Abraham." She keeps the covenant in faith and is a believer in the pre-Christian sense. She had a spirit of infirmity and was (in Jesus' own words) one "whom Satan has bound...for eighteen years"— a reference not just to this woman's sickness. Though not possessed by a demonic entity, the woman in this story was clearly oppressed and suffering acutely from this spirit of infirmity, whether it afflicted her anatomy or just loitered around to vandalize her life. Either way, she wanted to be free. If this covenant-keeping daughter of Abraham could host a spirit of infirmity for eighteen years, couldn't any believer be a target of demons?

Jesus didn't haltingly protest, "Wait, you're a believer, you can't have a demon." No, instead He declared freedom, deliverance, and healing. First, He proclaimed her to be loosed from the spirit of infirmity, and then He laid His hands upon her and she was healed. No matter how it is viewed, this "Christian" woman needed help to receive her freedom from a demonic assault against her.

In the case of the woman with the issue of blood, the demonic oppression had been present for some time, leading us to believe that some open door had allowed it permission to harass her. This type of demonic assault could be said to have been initiated through invitation; that is, the women had some issue in her life that had "invited" or "allowed" the demonic opportunity to stir up her sickness. On the other hand, demonic efforts to destroy the believer are not limited solely to those places where we have allowed them access. At other times, the enemy seeks to attack us through what may be described as intrusion, whereby, without the presence of either intentional or unintentional rebellion or sin, the enemy initiates a destructive attack against the believer. When open doors have given invitation to the enemy, we tend to describe the process of obtaining freedom as deliverance. However, when the enemy seems to intrude into the life of a believer, we often refer to the process of obtaining freedom as spiritual warfare. In such cases, the same authority that brings freedom from demonic oppression will put an end to the demonic intrusion.

In today's society, it is not uncommon to see occult activity paraded before us, either via the evening news or through demands for equal *religious* freedom. Satanism, witchcraft, Wicca, and other occult enterprises are active and unashamed to be identified. Many unbelievers are heavily oppressed by these and other satanic groups or influences, and some have wholly surrendered to them. The impact of demonic oppression is straightforward and easily discernible in some cases, but it also manifests in more devious, insidious ways through public recognition of these trends. Make no mistake: though not publicly stated, groups rooted in the demonic are determined to destroy the Church and tear down individual believers, for this is Satan's avowed agenda.

The men from the tombs in Matthew 8 are evidence of this type of covert attack against believers. Verse 28 describes these demon-possessed men as so fierce that no one could pass by their area. Another biblical example of the enemy's intent to destroy God's people is when King Saul was demonically influenced to throw his spear at David to kill him.[27] The intention of demonic forces, even though they may be operating through unbelievers ignorant of their devices, is to harm, hinder, and halt Christ's followers.

One Halloween several years ago, a well-known revelatory minister was staying in our home. The entire family had retired for the night, and everything seemed to be quiet until Michael was awakened around 1:00 A.M. by his mother pounding at the bedroom door. In a panic, she explained that Bill had awakened in a state of near-suffocation and was still struggling to breathe. Michael immediately went to the bedroom where their prophetic friend was staying, but before he could even lift his hand to knock, the door opened, and the guest, awake and fully dressed, said, "I've already taken care of the witches; now let's see about your dad." He hastened across the hall and prayed for Bill, who was instantly able to breathe freely again. Later, the guest explained that the Lord had awakened him and shown him that a group of witches was praying for Bill's death. He had gone in the spirit (similar to what Obadiah described Elijah doing in 1 Kings 18) and come against them, exercising God's authority over the demonic realm. He knew that when he prayed for Bill, the healing would come. We have never forgotten this incident, and anytime since, when we're under demonic attack, it reminds us that God already knows the situation and has already provided the means for us to overcome.

While believers continue to debate whether they can be possessed or just oppressed, God's Word says that our adversary, the devil, is a cunning and wily foe. We must not allow him access through any chink in our armor.

CHAPTER 4

WHO ARE OUR ALLIES?

Before diving into a discussion of the ministry of deliverance directly, it might be helpful to recognize that we are not alone in our battle. The first section of this book is intended to help us identify who our enemy is and how the demonic realm operates; however, these dark spiritual forces are not the only beings engaged in the conflict that surrounds us. Since we are involved in a spiritual battle with spiritual enemies, it seems only fitting that we should also have spiritual allies. As we discovered in Ephesians 6:12, our enemy is an organized opponent whose ranks include principalities, powers, rulers of darkness, and spiritual hosts of wickedness. This knowledge alone could lead us to a feeling that the battle may be too great and the odds stacked too high against us, but God has not left us alone to confront this darkness. Speaking of the unseen heavenly spiritual beings that stand together with us to confront the darkness, the author of Hebrews wrote:

> *Are they not all ministering spirits sent forth to minister for those who will inherit salvation?*
> —*Hebrews 1:14* NKJV

This passage seems to indicate that each of us, who have become inheritors of salvation, not only have the capability of ministering in the area of deliverance as the remainder of this book will make clear, but we also have the support of spiritual allies who have been assigned not merely to minister to us, but also to "minister for" us. While this army is not at our command, but rather takes its order from God, He has clearly established that they will join us in engaging the enemy in battle on our behalf.

The heavenly army that joins with us has an organizational structure that is equal to (or perhaps more appropriately, superior to) the ranks of the demonic world. While we have no individual scripture describing the heavenly ranks in the way that Ephesians 6 describes the demonic order, there is sufficient evidence throughout the Word of God to establish this fact with certainty. Consider one of the clearest spiritual warfare scenarios described in scripture when Daniel prays and the demonic principalities seek to hinder the answer to his prayer. This story provides one of our first absolute clues that the angelic realm is also engaged in the battle and that it has sufficient structure to fight well and overcome the enemy.

> *Then he said, "Do you know why I have come to you? And now I must return to fight with the prince of Persia; and when I have gone forth, indeed the prince of Greece will come. But I will tell you what is noted in the Scripture of Truth. (No one upholds me against these, except Michael your prince.)"*
> —*Daniel 10:20–21* NKJV

An angel, perhaps even Gabriel, had been engaged in battle with the demonic prince of Persia to bring the answer to Daniel's prayer, and Daniel's prince (verse 13 describes him as one of the chief princes)—Michael—came alongside to ensure that the answer was delayed no longer. From these verses, it seems that when rank is matched against rank (demonic prince versus heavenly prince), the light of God will always prevail.

If we have allies who are organized in rank and provide more than a fitting match against their demonic counterparts, then it could be helpful to identify who they are. While we have a tendency to label all of heaven's spiritual beings as angels, this does not appear to be an accurate description. For a better understanding, consider the following list of heavenly spiritual beings found in scripture:

- Cherubim (Ezekiel 10:3–8)
- Seraphim (Isaiah 6:2)
- Heavenly watchers (Daniel 4:13)
- Heavenly creatures (Ezekiel 1:5–6, 10; Revelation 4:6–7)
- Heavenly lights (James 1:17; Acts 20:8)
- Heavenly hosts (Luke 2:13–14)
- The cloud of witnesses (Hebrews 12:1)

While some of these heavenly beings are mentioned only briefly in Scripture, it clearly seems that there is more than a single generic rank of angels. Scripture is filled with examples of these heavenly beings, at times called angels and at times completely undesignated, serving and assisting God's people. It was heavenly beings who attempted to stop Balaam from going astray in Numbers 22 and who released Peter from prison in Acts 12, and these are only two of many scriptural examples.

Clearly, we have allies who assist us, and the passage referenced in Daniel alone supports the fact that they participate in the spiritual warfare in which we are engaged. However, lest we underestimate their role, it is important to remember that these supernatural beings are involved in many activities that help us as believers while we walk through this life. The examples from Scripture are too numerous to list, but consider these few functions that they perform:

- Giving direction/delivering messages (such as the instructions provided to Gideon in Judges 6 or the announcement made to the shepherds in Luke 2)
- Releasing judgment (such as making Lot's attackers blind in Genesis 19 or making Zacharias mute in Luke 1)
- Going before to prepare the way (such as finding Isaac's wife in Genesis 24:7, 40)
- Protecting God's people (such as preserving Daniel in the lions' den in Daniel 6)
- Strengthening God's servants (such as providing Elijah food as he fled Jezebel in 1 Kings 19 or strengthening Jesus in the garden in Luke 22:43)
- Gathering the harvest of souls (such as in the Parable of the Tares in Matthew 13)
- Taking physical action in the earth (such as rolling the stone from the tomb in Matthew 28, stirring the waters at the Pool of Bethesda in John 5, or breaking Peter's chains in Acts 12)
- Guarding things (such as those assigned to the Garden of Eden in Genesis 3:24)
- Encouraging God's people (such as that done by the great cloud of witnesses in Hebrews 12)

These spiritual beings are powerful allies, moving and acting in an invisible realm that exists all around us. While many of the battles they fight and the tasks they accomplish may never be known to us, they are always preparing the way for the freedom of God's children. As we begin to examine the ministry of deliverance, it is important to know that we are not alone. Certainly, God is on our side, and through Him we can overcome any demonic assault, but in addition, He has also commissioned His ministering spirits to aid us in this fight.

Finally, it is important to consider one last point. Now that we know who our enemy is and we recognize that we have allies in the fight, it is also significant that we recognize who we are. The Word of God declares that you are:

- Born of incorruptible seed (1 Peter 1:23)
- A child of God (1 John 3:2–3)
- An heir of God (Galatians 4:6–7)
- A disciple of Jesus (John 8:31–32)
- The salt of the earth (Matthew 5:13)
- A light to the world (Matthew 5:14–16)
- Valuable (Matthew 10:29–31)
- The temple of God (1 Corinthians 3:16–17)
- A new creation (2 Corinthians 5:17)
- The body of Christ (1 Corinthians 12:27)
- A partaker of consolation (2 Corinthians 1:7)
- An overcomer (1 John 4:4)
- Strong (2 Corinthians 12:9–10)
- Not ashamed (Romans 1:16)
- A branch of the vine (John 15:5)
- Special, chosen, royal, and priestly (1 Peter 2:9)
- An ambassador (2 Corinthians 5:20)
- The righteousness of God (2 Corinthians 5:21)
- Bold (Hebrews 4:16)
- Capable of great things (Philippians 4:13)
- A friend of God (John 15:15)
- Content (Philippians 4:11–13)

Considering who you are and the support that God has clearly provided for you as a believer, it would be foolish to think anything less than that He wants you to be free and for you to freely give away what you have received.[28]

Remedy: Freedom Through Deliverance

SECTION TWO
THE REMEDY

In the first section, we examined who the enemy is and what he can do. To stop there would give Satan unnecessary glory. It is essential that we now explore how to thwart his plans.

Efforts to stand up to the enemy are usually called *spiritual warfare*, while the specific ministry employed to free an individual from the enemy is termed *deliverance*. The primary topic of this book is the ministry of deliverance.

Section Two is not designed to offer a formula or procedure for ministering to an individual, but to give basic insights into the elements necessary to receive freedom and to help others walk in that freedom. This section is titled "*Remedy*" because it addresses how an individual can overcome or "remedy" the demonic attack that has targeted him or her for destruction.

Breaking free from demonic attack isn't particularly easy. It requires work, understanding, and most importantly, a solid foundation in God's Word. The scriptural principles we discuss here are not intended as a guidebook for dealing with specific problems, but they focus on a broad foundation of biblical principles, which will help an individual gain spiritual freedom, regardless of the problem. Whether the issue is Satanism, witchcraft, occultism, drugs, alcohol, or anything else that disrupts proper godly and balanced behavior, the following principles lay a basic foundation for freedom from demonic attacks on believers.

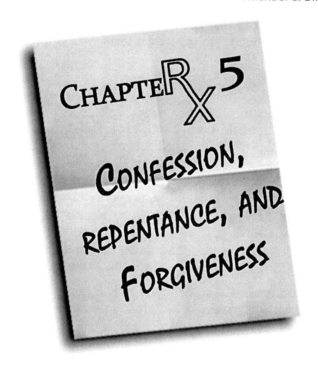

CHAPTER X 5

CONFESSION, REPENTANCE, AND FORGIVENESS

Regardless of the type of ongoing demonic attack a person is facing, it is happening because the person has been opened to it, either knowingly or unknowingly. In order for a person to experience true freedom from demonic oppression, the root cause must be identified and addressed. If a person is experiencing a great deal of oppression that just won't let up, somewhere an open door has given the enemy a foothold in that individual's life. The initial step in deliverance ministry is to deal with sin and disobedience; however, it is very important to remember that not all oppression a person faces is the result of sin. Some oppression occurs because, like a disease, it literally runs in the family. Certain demonic influences can be passed down through the bloodlines. Traumatic events experienced as a child can also open the door to demonic activity. Confession, repentance, and forgiveness have a vital role to play in preparing the way for a person's freedom, no matter the type or intensity of oppression.

Confession

Confession is an integral part of every believer's daily walk from the outset of his or her relationship with Jesus Christ. The Word is clear that confession is crucial to our salvation experience. We must *confess* with our mouth and believe in our heart in order to be saved (Romans 10:9). To put it simply, confession is an act of verbal acknowledgment that brings us into agreement or covenant with God. This element of our Christian walk is so significant that Jesus Himself declares that if we confess Him before men, He will confess us before God. Conversely, if we deny Him before men, He will deny us before God (Matthew 10:33).

Just as confession is significant in receiving salvation, it is also extremely significant in gaining freedom from demonic oppression.

> *If we confess our sins, He is faithful and just to forgive us our sins and to cleanse us from all unrighteousness.*
> —*1 John 1:9* NKJV

In order to find freedom, any opening for demonic attack we have given the enemy must be sealed. Confession is the first step in closing that opening. When we confess, or acknowledge, where we have fallen short, God is faithful not only to forgive us, but also to cleanse us. Forgiveness is necessary for our redemption and reconciliation to God, but cleansing slams shut the doors we have opened to the enemy.

Those seeking freedom from demonic assault must be willing to examine their hearts and allow the Lord to reveal any sin that has given the enemy place in their lives. However, merely recognizing that sin exists or has existed in their lives is not enough: they must confess and acknowledge that sin to God. Confession often is a private matter between the individual and God, but in the context of deliverance, it can also involve confession before others.

> *Confess your trespasses to one another, and pray for one another, that you may be healed. The effective, fervent prayer of a righteous man avails much.*
>
> —*James 5:16* NKJV

Confession before God gives Him access to forgive and cleanse, but as the preceding scripture indicates, when we confess our trespasses to one another, we can be healed and minister to one another. The Greek word *iaomai* (ee-ah'-om'ahee), translated as "healing" in this verse, conveys the message of being cured or made whole. Those subjected to demonic attack need restoration of what the enemy stole from them. Confessing to trustworthy ministers the sins that initially caused the oppression can be an effective step toward freedom and wholeness.

Obviously, such confession requires trust on the part of the individual making himself or herself vulnerable. In addition, there is a serious responsibility on the part of those hearing such disclosure. The rewards of this type of accountability can be tremendous. Some of the enemy's most preferred and effective tools to keep people in bondage are secrecy and shame.

Repentance

Confession opens the door to healing, but the process cannot be completed without true repentance, which means to truly change and go another direction (as implied by the Hebrew word *metanoia* (met-an'-oy-ah), meaning a change of mind or reversal of decision. While confession acknowledges before God (and/or humanity) what the enemy has used to hold someone captive, repentance ensures by a combination of word and deed that such ground is not readily given up again. Confession admits, "I'm guilty; I'm sorry," but repentance redirects and reforms an individual's set course.

> *Now I rejoice, not that you were made sorry, but that your sorrow led to repentance. For you were made sorry in a godly manner, that you might suffer loss from us in nothing.*
> —*2 Corinthians 7:9* NKJV

Confession and repentance lead to change, and change makes certain that freedom is received and maintained. If confession and repentance are not consistently practiced, the freedom initially gained may be lost later, hence the person quickly returns to bondage.

Repentance compels change in attitude and behavior; it demands determination, for once a person has opened the door to even the smallest sin, the enemy rushes in like a flood. The destructive habits that the enemy produces in an individual can be difficult to break and need persistence, and sometimes assistance, to be overcome. Repentance is only lip service if one does not consciously work at changing negative habits—and God certainly is not mocked. He knows when we are not being honest with Him, when we have no intention of actually changing our destructive behavior.

However, it is important to remember that when a given habit leads to a certain course of action or set of circumstances, it does not always mean that a person has returned to bondage. Rather, it may be a warning that he or she must make further effort to maintain freedom. (A more detailed examination of this topic is found in Chapter 8.)

Forgiveness

Despite our willingness to confess and repent, we might still encounter certain hindrances to overcoming demonic attacks. The greatest barrier to freedom, one that is often overlooked by well-meaning believers, lies in our own unforgiving hearts.

Jesus stated unequivocally that if we do not forgive, we cannot be forgiven.

> *"For if you forgive men their trespasses, your heavenly Father will also forgive you. But if you do not forgive men their trespasses, neither will your Father forgive your trespasses."*
> —*Matthew 6:14–15* NKJV

This principle is recorded not once but multiple times in the New Testament. Given this scriptural framework, possibly the two greatest blocks to receiving God's fullness are unwillingness to forgive oneself and unwillingness to forgive others.

Forgiving Ourselves

Sometimes, it can seem holier for us to forgive others but then continue harboring deep unforgiveness toward ourselves. The importance of the commandment to forgive ourselves in the same way we would forgive others is expressed by Jesus Himself when He is questioned about the greatest commandment:

> *Then one of the scribes came, and having heard them reasoning together, perceiving that He had answered them well, asked Him, "Which is the first commandment of all?" Jesus answered him, "The first of all the commandments is: 'Hear, O Israel, the LORD our God, the LORD is one. And you shall love the LORD your God with all your heart, with all your soul, with all your mind, and with all your strength.' This is the first commandment. And the second, like it, is this: 'You shall love your neighbor as yourself.' There is no other commandment greater than these."*
> —*Mark 12:28–31* NKJV

This passage deals as much with our relationship with ourselves as it does with our relationship with God and others. Jesus proclaims, "You shall love your neighbor as yourself." In other words, Jesus would not have us value ourselves any less or have us experience any less of His love than we value others and know He values them. He loves them, and us, enough to die on a cross to reconcile all humanity to Himself. We *must* forgive our own trespasses if we seek to be truly free from any demonic toehold in our lives.

So, one of the barriers to freedom from demonic oppression is failing to forgive ourselves. This failure often arises not from unwillingness, but rather from a lack of understanding of its necessity. We tend to judge ourselves by a stricter standard than the one we use to judge others. We must not only be obedient to God's Word, but we must be recipients of His promises, as well. If God is faithful to forgive us, who are we to do any less?

Forgiving versus Forgetting

Since we were created in the image of a forgiving God, we inherited this forgiving nature in our spiritual DNA. Not only has the enemy deceived us by masking God's forgiving nature, but he has gone for the jugular by convincing many believers that they have not been forgiven because they have not forgotten. Forgiving does not entail forgetting.

Just because we continue to remember our own or another's sin does not mean we have not forgiven or been forgiven by God. Forgiveness is a decision, an act of the will; it is not an emotion and has nothing to do with memory. It is that simple.

Satan is a liar.[29] He continually seeks to confuse us about forgiveness. We must place our trust in God's Word and not in the enemy's lies. It doesn't matter what we've done or what's been done to us, because God will forgive *all* sins, except blaspheming the Holy Spirit—and someone seeking help to be free from the enemy's hold is extremely unlikely to be guilty of that sin.

The following example illustrates the connection between forgiveness and deliverance. Sadly, a common root cause of demonic oppression is physical and/or sexual abuse endured as a child. Often, the abuse cycle has continued throughout the person's life. In one such case, our team had been ministering to an individual for some time with limited success because the root of the problem had not yet been identified. By revelation and the gift of discerning of spirits, it was apparent that demonic forces were cast out. However, this individual's life did not seem to improve. During one session, after much gentle, loving discussion, the individual opened up, and all the physical and sexual abuse she had experienced (which included several family members) began to surface. When asked how she felt toward her abusers, she conveyed intense dislike bordering on hatred. The team then began a lengthy examination of forgiveness, and after a season of prayer, discussion, and communicating the truth from God's Word, the individual finally decided to forgive. That decision was a choice and not a momentary feeling, and it was somewhat effective. Ministry resumed, but there was still limited success, with no evidence of transformation. The individual remained downcast, depressed, and suicidal.

One problem remained—forgiveness was not yet complete. Although the individual had chosen to forgive her abusers, she had not forgiven herself. When the team gingerly broached this issue, they encountered staunch resistance. But once they were able to show that this was a biblical command, it was accepted and acted upon. The results were phenomenal. The woman's countenance was transfigured. An upbeat attitude began to supplant the weary, downcast nature. Depression and suicide, which had haunted her for most of her life, became a thing of the past. As her bitterness died, this individual's life was transformed. Deliverance had been progressing incrementally all along, but the final and lasting transformation came after choosing to forgive others and herself.

Now, this woman certainly did not immediately forget all the wrongs she had endured. In fact, to date, those memories still linger. However, when she recognized that her entrapment lay not in the memories of what had been done to her (which she could not change), but in her heart attitude toward her abusers and herself (which she could change), she found a key to her freedom. Forgiveness did not mean forgetting or restoring relationships with her abusers. It did mean releasing the mental, emotional, and spiritual captivity wrought by bitterness, anger, and hatred and also relinquishing the destructive attitudes that had festered since the abuse.

Longing to rewrite the past also hampers forgiving or receiving forgiveness. The past cannot be changed; we can't do anything about it. We may worry about how others perceive it. We may wallow in what would have, should have, or could have been. We can even lie about how it really was. But we cannot change it.

Where we have failed God in the past, we must simply ask Him for forgiveness, believe His Word is true, and recognize that His forgiveness is ours for the taking. We must embrace God's forgiveness...despite our memories. Where others have failed us, we must choose to forgive them, believe it is a decision and not an emotion, and move on despite our memories.

Simple Beginnings

Unconfessed sin, false repentance, and unforgiveness can keep us in the fire of demonic attack. Freedom begins when we address these areas. Though they may seem elementary to some, it is amazing how quickly we can be led to forget them during hard times. No monumental revelation or vast and glorious theological point serves to improve this formula: the Gospel remains simple and effective despite our best efforts (and those of the enemy) to make it complicated.

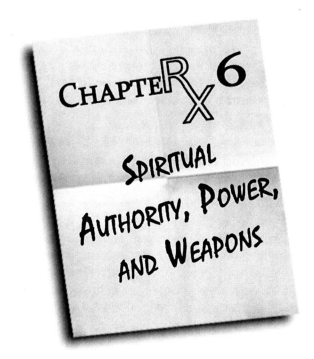

CHAPTER 6

SPIRITUAL AUTHORITY, POWER, AND WEAPONS

The preceding chapter focused on the initial steps one can take to find freedom from oppression. This chapter builds on that foundation and will benefit both those seeking freedom and those ministering to them. Ministry cannot be based on a formula; however, the following scriptural foundation can address any kind of spiritual bondage.

God's Word declares that every believer is a minister. In Ephesians 4:12, the role of the fivefold minister is to equip the saints (believers) for the work of the ministry. While not every believer is called to actual deliverance ministry, every believer does have the capability of ministering in the area of deliverance. Our contemporary mind-set considers ministry a full- or part-time job, but scripturally, ministry simply means fulfilling what the Word of God commands. Every believer is not realistically expected to engage in deliverance as a vocation; however, on the other hand, every believer is called, according to God's Word, to engage in the *work of the ministry*. In other words, everything needed to minister deliverance is present in the life of every believer who is willing to make him or herself available for the Lord to prepare and use. Scripture confirms this in several different places:

- "Whatever you ask..." (John 16:23 NKJV)
- "If two of you agree..." (Matthew 18:19 NKJV)
- "Behold, I give you the authority..." (Luke 10:19 NKJV)

God has given believers authority and power in His name, along with every spiritual weapon necessary to receive and minister freedom. The work of the ministry is not entrusted only to apostles, prophets, evangelists, pastors, or teachers, but *each one* of us—every disciple of Jesus—has a measure of grace according to Christ's gift.[30]

In addition to equipping the saints for the work of ministry, the role of the fivefold minister is to edify the body of Christ so that we *all* come into unity, the fullness of our calling, and spiritual maturity.[31] Fivefold ministers may have responsibilities that differ from others, but they don't have special abilities or are more capable in and of themselves. What sharply distinguishes fivefold ministers is their level of favor with God and humanity and also an understanding of the anointing.

Both anointing and favor are divine gifts that we cannot humanly manufacture. Simply put, anointing reflects the degree of God's power and authority functioning in an individual's life, while God's favor can be demonstrated by the presence of gifts and the ability to minister successfully in specific areas. Favor with people is granted by God and results in a marked difference in how others receive ministry. Favor and anointing afford true fivefold and vocational ministers greater effectiveness in ministering and increase their spiritual impact and scope.

Authority

Believers can accomplish the acts described in God's Word only with God's authority. Though we face an enemy who is strong and powerful, every believer has the opportunity to walk in authority over him. The primary problem is the believers' failure to recognize the authority available to them.

Jesus describes the single greatest grant of authority found in the New Testament.

> *"Most assuredly, I say to you, he who believes in Me, the works that I do he will do also; and greater works than these he will do, because I go to My Father. And whatever you ask in My name, that I will do, that the Father may be glorified in the Son. If you ask anything in My name, I will do it."*
>
> —*John 14:12–14 NKJV*

This promise is one of the most remarkable in God's Word; however, like most of God's promises, it is conditional. Jesus Himself promises that we can do all the works He did (and even greater works), but we must first believe in Him. Anything that we ask will be done, but we must first learn what it means to ask in His name. These words testify that a tremendous amount of authority has been granted believers. Jesus performed some amazing feats: He turned water into wine, made blind eyes see and deaf ears hear; He cleansed lepers and multiplied loaves and fishes; He healed the sick, raised the dead, and drove out demons.

While the next chapter will more fully examine how we become recipients of the authority Jesus offered here, it is important at this stage to understand the significance of the words "in My name." For too long, the Church has simply assumed that using the five-word phrase "in the name of Jesus" was akin to waving a magic wand and that by saying those words, it was supposed to mean we got whatever we asked for, instead of realizing that functioning in the name of Jesus was all about deepening our relationship with Him.

Luke also records Jesus' giving believers authority.

> *"Behold, I give you the authority to trample on serpents and scorpions, and over all the power of the enemy, and nothing shall by any means hurt you."*
>
> —*Luke 10:19 NKJV*

Here again, Jesus is granting believers authority over the forces of darkness. Serpents and scorpions denote demons and devils, and believers have been given authority to put them under their feet—not just demons and devils but *all* the power of the enemy. The word *all* doesn't leave out anything.

This authority is powerful and offers tremendous supernatural protection from the enemy's plans. For example, Bill was once ministering to a man skilled in various martial arts. During the course of ministry, this man stood up, took a martial arts posture, and began threatening the ministry team. Although this was potentially a very dangerous situation, Bill wielded his authority in the Lord and ordered the man in Jesus' name to sit and be quiet. The man immediately went rigid and fell backward onto the floor, where he remained for the rest of the ministry time. Knowing the authority we have in Christ averted the potential danger. Interestingly enough, this individual later became one of Bill's most helpful ministry assistants. While we are walking in divine authority, we are also walking in divine protection from the enemy. Satan's arsenal is neutralized.

Power

Power is given by the Holy Spirit for purposes of upholding the authority in which we walk. The difference between power and authority is found in the classic example of the weight lifter and the policeman. Under the right conditions, both of them can stop a moving vehicle. The weight lifter, if properly trained and conditioned, has enough power to lift the wheels off the ground and prevent the car from moving. On the other hand, though a police officer may be unable to lift as much weight, his authority can stop the same vehicle. By simply raising his hand and commanding, "Stop!" the police officer accomplishes the same thing the weight lifter did with less effort. He is able to stop the vehicle, not in his own strength, but because the law of the land gives him the right to do so and requires every citizen to obey. The officer's authority is enhanced because he carries a weapon in a holster at his side, and he has an army of police officers back at department headquarters to assist him.

God's Word has not granted you authority without the power to enforce and enhance it. Everything created is subject to the Word of God—including Satan and the demonic world. The hosts of heaven stand waiting to help fight against the enemy, and God's Word specifically gives us the power to do it. Jesus promised in Luke 24:49 that when He ascended to heaven, He would send the Father's promise, and we would be endued with power from on high. Paul also confirmed the power available to the believer.

> *"But you shall receive power when the Holy Spirit has come upon you; and you shall be witnesses to Me in Jerusalem, and in all Judea and Samaria, and to the end of the earth."*
> —*Acts 1:8* NKJV

This is the same power Jesus used in His deliverance ministry.

> *"And if I cast out demons by Beelzebub, by whom do your sons cast them out? Therefore they shall be your judges. But if I cast out demons by the Spirit of God, surely the kingdom of God has come upon you."*
> —*Matthew 12:27–28* NKJV

Jesus cast out demons by the Spirit of God, with the very same power you have. This power is the Holy Spirit's presence in your life, enabling you to accomplish what you have been offered the authority to do.

Weapons

The gifts and weapons Jesus gave us work only because the Holy Spirit directly empowers them. To understand their use in ministry, it is important to understand the difference between the weapons and the tools that God supplies. Weapons are the implements used to convey power, just like the police officer's gun; tools are the methods we use to accomplish what God has given us to do.

This book isn't meant to provide a detailed analysis of the tools available for deliverance ministry, which may include questionnaires, lists of commonly encountered demonic strongholds, interviewing methods, and more. However, weapons are scripturally based and must be used no matter what type of ministry we're doing.

Prayer

The most powerful and effective weapon available to the believer is prayer. Prayer is not a posture, a position, or an eloquent speech. It is not determined by education or the ability to be heard over a crowd. God speaks your language. No one has to pray in biblical King James English. Prayer does not entail reciting sundry religious clichés or barraging God with instructions. Simply put, prayer means communication with God in a way that seeks His will in our life or in another's.

Praying with command and authority is an invaluable principle of prayer that is often overlooked. It proclaims the spiritual authority of God's Word and commands demonic forces to honor and obey that authority. Jesus employed this type of prayer nearly every time He freed people from demonic forces. Also, He often prepared for ministry by spending the whole night in the mountains alone in prayer. Then, when the time came to actually touch an individual's life, Jesus exercised command and authority. Examples of this are numerous throughout the Gospels.

For instance, when Jesus confronted the two demon-possessed men among the tombs in Matthew 8, He simply commanded, "Go," and the demons departed. In Luke 4, again Jesus merely orders obedience, and it is done:

> But Jesus rebuked him, saying, "Be quiet, and come out of him!" And when the demon had thrown him in their midst, it came out of him and did not hurt him.
>
> —Luke 4:35 NKJV

Jesus exemplified that, when dealing with the demonic realm on earth, the believer has absolute authority to command obedience. Present-day examples of this authority abound and function both in context of commanding the demonic to depart and in commanding it to comply. While traveling and teaching in Africa, Michael has noticed, on numerous occasions, that ministry seems to be a bit more physically intense. On one occasion, while observing a local African ministry team, a number of those receiving deliverance were thrashing about on the floor. One in particular began to roll violently toward the door with Michael directly in her path. The typical response to such a situation by the local team had been to have someone hold the individual down. On this occasion, no one was prepared to stop the individual, so Michael simply commanded her to: "Be still! In the name of Jesus," and she immediately ceased rolling and went limp on the floor.

Name of Jesus

For the believer, the ability to command the enemy comes through the use of Jesus' name.

> *"And whatever you ask in My name, that I will*
> *do, that the Father may be glorified in the Son.*
> *If you ask anything in My name, I will do it."*
> —*John 14:13–14* NKJV

If Jesus could say, "Go," and demons departed, then every believer has the ability to command, "Go in the name of Jesus," and see equal results. The name of Jesus is one of the most powerful weapons of our warfare.

Using Jesus' name is powerful; however, simply saying "Jesus" doesn't always carry authority—after all, many people invoke His name as a swear word. We as believers, the servants of God, carry His authority and don't actually have to speak Jesus' name in order to use it. In ancient times, when a king sent out his servants, they were empowered to act "in the name of the king." This power did not demand the addition of the words "in the king's name" to their every request, command, or action; rather, the use of the king's name meant that, as his servants, what they did or said on his behalf had the same force and effect as though he himself were present. As Ephesians 4 saints mature in the ways of the Holy Spirit, all believers have been given access to use the name of the King of kings, and what we do or say (as long as we are walking in the Spirit) carries authority. Kings throughout history have sent ambassadors to conduct their business. The King of kings, being omnipresent and resident within every believer, stands with us whenever we invoke the authority of His name. Our authority to use Jesus' name is inherent in our relationship with the King Himself; thus, the deeper the relationship, the greater the authority. We must understand that just as in ancient times, if the character and actions of the servant do not conform to the nature of the king, then authority that would otherwise be present would be lost, whether or not the name was actually verbalized.

Even though we don't have to verbalize Jesus' name to use it, speaking His name is still very important in ministry and prayer, as Scripture clearly demonstrates. One biblical example is the account of the slave girl in Acts.

> *Now it happened, as we went to prayer, that a certain slave girl possessed with a spirit of divination met us, who brought her masters much profit by fortune-telling. This girl followed Paul and us, and cried out, saying, "These men are the servants of the Most High God, who proclaim to us the way of salvation." And this she did for many days. But Paul, greatly annoyed, turned and said to the spirit, "I command you in the name of Jesus Christ to come out of her." And he came out that very hour.*
>
> —Acts 16:16–18 NKJV

Jesus' name is above every other name, and at His name every knee will bow.[32] So, when we glorify Jesus' name through a walk consistent with His character and nature and when we physically speak His name, we wield a mighty weapon against the forces of darkness.

Blood of Jesus

An equally effective weapon of warfare is Christ's blood. Jesus' shed blood is a continual reminder to the enemy that his best-laid plans failed. In the moment he perceived to be his ultimate triumph, the crucifixion of Jesus, Satan met his ultimate defeat. Jesus' innocent blood was spilled as the perfect sacrifice for sin and restored the opportunity for human relationship with God. Each time Jesus' blood is mentioned in the presence of demonic spirits, they are forced to recall the humiliation they suffered when their plans went awry and their doom was sealed. The terror the mere mentioning of Jesus' blood inspires among demonic spirits is heartening; yet, to truly use Jesus' blood effectively as a weapon, we must understand its biblical basis.

> *And they overcame him by the blood of the Lamb
> and by the word of their testimony, and they did
> not love their lives to the death.*
> —*Revelation 12:11* NKJV

The blood of the Lamb (Jesus) is a weapon used to overcome the great dragon, Satan, the serpent of old.[33] By the shedding of Jesus' innocent blood, the devil was defeated at Calvary, and thus when he is reminded of the blood he is reminded of his defeat. If Jesus' blood is sufficient to overcome the devil himself, then it definitely is an effective weapon against his demonic forces.

Word of God

One easily overlooked weapon is the direct use of God's Word. Memorization of Scripture is powerful and effective. The Word that proceeds from the mouth of the Lord will accomplish its purpose.

> *So shall My word be that goes forth from My
> mouth; it shall not return to Me void, but it shall
> accomplish what I please, and it shall prosper in
> the thing for which I sent it.*
> —*Isaiah 55:11* NKJV

It is powerful to have someone read from the Word while ministry is taking place. During one ministry session, Bill learned that not only is Scripture an effective weapon when proclaimed boldly against our adversary, but the Bible (as a book) itself can also be useful. While ministering to a young woman, Bill placed his Bible across her hands, which were resting on her knees. When he did, she immediately asked, "Would you take that book off my hands, please?" Recognizing that something unique was taking place, Bill refused and told her that if she wanted it off, she would have to remove it herself. After a few moments of debate, she insisted that she didn't want to remove it because if she did, it would ruin their faith. Bill, unwilling to give in to this demonic challenge, again refused to remove the Bible. Finally, the young woman (or more particularly, the demonic entity working through her) acceded and said, "Would you move the book, please? It is burning my hands." While the Bible does not identify itself in its book form as an effective weapon, this experience reveals that God's Word, in any form, is powerful.

Anointing Oil

Anointing oil is another potent weapon in ministry, although it is mentioned only briefly in Scripture. Oil, in and of itself, is insignificant, but when it has been prayed over and consecrated to the Lord, it can wreak damage on darkness. Oil represents the Holy Spirit's presence and the anointing. In the Old Testament, it was an integral part of the furnishings of the tabernacle. In Exodus 25:6, it kept the flames of the tabernacle lamps alive and was also used for anointing. In Leviticus 8:10–12, it was used for anointing both the tabernacle and the priest. In the New Testament, anointing with oil is connected with healing ministry and is also a strong weapon in deliverance (itself a form of healing). Perhaps the most famous scripture outlining the use of anointing oil is in the book of James.

> *Is anyone among you sick? Let him call for the elders of the church, and let them pray over him, anointing him with oil in the name of the Lord. And the prayer of faith will save the sick, and the Lord will raise him up. And if he has committed sins, he will be forgiven.*
> —James 5:14–15 NKJV

Another passage that indicates Jesus approved the use of anointing oil and probably instructed His disciples in its use is in the book of Mark.

> *And they cast out many demons, and anointed with oil many who were sick, and healed them.*
> —Mark 6:13 NKJV

While Scripture doesn't directly connect anointing oil to deliverance ministry, it certainly does so indirectly. As seen in James 5:14, those who are sick are to be anointed with oil, and verse 15 goes on to say that the "prayer of faith will save the sick..." The Greek word *arrhostos* (ar'-hroce-tos) translated as "sick" is used of any who are tired, worn down, or feeble, while the word *sozo* (sode'-zo) translated as "save" means to save, deliver, or protect.[34] Oil has proved beneficial in present-day application, as well, as demonstrated in the following story.

In ministering to a young woman who was heavily involved in the occult and had willingly participated in several human sacrifices, our team ultimately found it difficult to get her to commit to the deliverance process. On a few occasions after ministry began, she actually jumped up and fled the room. Wanting to help her, the ministry team continued to work with her. The final time Bill saw her for ministry, she was sitting in front of his desk weeping. Bill instructed one of the men to put anointing oil on his hand and place it on her head. When he did, she screamed loudly, fell to the floor, and lay there screaming for quite a while. Finally, a particularly strong demonic entity surfaced, caused her to stand, and announced the woman was leaving. Bill's ministry assistant, experimenting with this new-found weapon, reached over and rubbed his oily hand on the doorknob to the only exit from the room. When the woman reached the door, she examined the knob carefully and tried to touch it several times. At last, in desperation, she gingerly gripped the doorknob with a bunch of tissue and escaped the room. Unfortunately, she never returned for further ministry. Although this situation could be viewed as a failure, the lesson learned about the power of anointing oil has been a significant help in setting many others free.

Binding and Loosing

God's Word establishes the principle of binding and loosing as a powerful weapon against demons.

"Assuredly, I say to you, whatever you bind on earth will be bound in heaven, and whatever you loose on earth will be loosed in heaven."
—*Matthew 18:18* NKJV

In a later chapter, we further discuss the principle of binding and loosing as it relates to spiritual warfare. Demonic entities must be present in the earthly realm to oppress individuals; because of this, believers can bind these demonic entities and order their activity to cease. Binding the enemy forces him to loose minds or emotions and allows the people under this intense oppression to think for themselves. Scripture and experience attest how crucial this principle is to deliverance ministry and beyond.

In the early days of ministry, before fully understanding how to use this weapon, Bill would frequently request aid from other men in restraining those receiving ministry. This was to keep them from hurting themselves. He learned by experience that this was not the most effective method and that it gave the enemy the opportunity to bring accusations against the ministry. One day while ministering to a young man who was about to get up from his folding chair and attack those ministering to him, Bill declared, "In the name of Jesus, I bind your hands to the sides of that chair." For the rest of the ministry session, the young man could not remove his hands from the chair. He continued trying to get up and actually ran around the room holding the chair against himself, but he was unable to release it. It is important to remember here that the demonic entity was controlling the young man's actions, not the young man himself. When the demonic presence was gone, the man was completely free to exercise his will to release the chair.

Binding and loosing is effectual both when commanding demonic entities to depart and when deliverance may not be the appropriate action. Occasionally, individuals may be so oppressed and confused that they can't clearly decide whether they actually want freedom or not. In this circumstance, it would be appropriate to bind the demonic entities from operating and command them to loose the people's minds, allowing the people a respite of peace and rest so they can choose to allow the Lord to act. Binding and loosing can open the door for the Lord to draw individuals to freedom.

Agreement

The biblical principle of agreement can be an excellent asset in spiritual warfare. Agreement not only concentrates the delivery of God's power, but also multiplies its effectiveness. Unfortunately, believers rarely actually agree. The primary scriptural basis for the principle of agreement is found in Matthew.

> *"Again I say to you that if two of you agree on earth concerning anything that they ask, it will be done for them by My Father in heaven."*
> —*Matthew 18:19* NKJV

In addition to the virtually unlimited favor God grants as a result of agreement, His Word states that when two or more come together in agreement, a tremendous increase in impact is released. Deuteronomy 32:30 testifies that, when the Lord is in charge, one can put a thousand to flight and two can put ten thousand to flight. Spiritual force increases exponentially when two or more individuals agree. Unfortunately, believers have not yet tapped in to the full manifestation of this power because we rarely arrive at actual agreement.

The weapon of agreement is based on being of one accord. Though believers often express agreement with a particular prayer or proclamation, all too often this is not actually true agreement. Commonly, the group of believers is mentally *assenting* that something is probably true without ever really *agreeing* that it is. Even when believers do agree, they are often violating the biblical principle by asking with the wrong motives. Every passage of Scripture must be taken in context with the rest of God's Word if we are to properly interpret it. In this case, the Word says that, when two agree, they can have whatever they ask, but we must always take note of how and why we ask.

> *You lust and do not have. You murder and covet and cannot obtain. You fight and war. Yet you do not have because you do not ask. You ask and do not receive, because you ask amiss, that you may spend it on your pleasures.*
> —James 4:2–3 NKJV

When we link this passage with Matthew 18, we realize our prayers may not be answered because we don't agree and because we are asking amiss. For agreement and asking principles to function, we must ask according to what God wants rather than what we want. Too often, our prayers are based on our human desires instead of God's heart. In order to properly use the weapon of agreement, we must go beyond a mental assent and find the mind of God for what we are asking. When these principles are applied, agreement will become a powerful weapon in the believer's arsenal.

The bottom line is that we be must be willing to use the weapons God has provided and not let fear inactivate us or expect someone else to do the job we've been called to do. All the authority, power, and weapons—the remedy Jesus won for us—are useless unless we are willing to use them.

The Source of Power and Authority

Power and authority are essential to a believer's ability to deal with the demonic. While the demonic world itself and the subject of deliverance are not without controversy, the source from which a believer draws their power and authority can be some of the most controversial and misunderstood topics in the Christian community. The first step to understanding power and authority in our lives is to recognize that we have often failed to distinguish between the two and subsequently failed to recognize that they come from two separate biblical sources. Authority will always supersede power, as previously indicated in the reference to Luke 10:19. So, what's the difference? The Greek word most commonly translated "power" is *dunamis* (doo'-nam-is), coming from the root word *dunamai* (doo'-nam-ahee). For all practical purposes, this term could be translated as ability, might, power, or strength. Power can be understood as strength or the ability to do something—specifically in our case, the ability to live a visible Christian life. The Greek word used most frequently for authority is *exousia* (ex-oo-see'-ah), and at its core this is the "right" to do something rather than the "ability." It can be seen as force, capacity, competency, mastery, or delegated influence. On the other hand, this word *exousia* most often translated as "authority" is also occasionally translated as "power," thus further complicating our inability to distinguish between the two.

Power is a gift received along with the Holy Spirit, and it grants to us the ability to live a Christian life—to be a witness. Authority is obtained as we draw near to the Father and walk in righteousness, giving us the "right" to change the atmosphere around us. By exercising the delegated influence received from relationship with the Father, we can "do" the work of the kingdom—heal the sick, raise the dead, cleanse the leper, and cast out demons.

> Then He called His twelve disciples together and gave them *power* and *authority over all demons*, and to cure diseases. He sent them to preach the kingdom of God and to heal the sick.
> —Luke 9:1–2 NKJV *(emphasis added)*

The Source of Power

Believers must harness a supernatural power of the Holy Spirit to deal with demons. According to John 14:26, the Holy Spirit is given as our teacher in spiritual matters, our helper, and our guide along the path of righteousness. He becomes the mouthpiece of God the Father, giving us instructions from God's Word and by that still, small voice He uses to speak directly to our hearts. In John 14:26, Jesus states that the Holy Spirit will be sent in His name both to teach us and to bring us into remembrance of what He said. The Holy Spirit also empowers by diverse gifts given as He chooses. Sometimes described as a second filling of the Holy Spirit, another aspect of the Holy Spirit's role in a believer's life is the baptism of the Holy Spirit.

> *When the Day of Pentecost had fully come, they were all with one accord in one place. And suddenly there came a sound from heaven, as of a rushing mighty wind, and it filled the whole house where they were sitting. Then there appeared to them divided tongues, as of fire, and one sat upon each of them. And they were all filled with the Holy Spirit and began to speak with other tongues, as the Spirit gave them utterance.*
>
> —Acts 2:1–4 NKJV

The filling with the Holy Spirit is designed to empower disciples to be witnesses.

> *"But you shall receive power when the Holy Spirit has come upon you; and you shall be witnesses to Me in Jerusalem, and in all Judea and Samaria, and to the end of the earth."*
>
> —Acts 1:8 NKJV

After the disciples were filled with the Holy Spirit, they immediately began to exercise power and boldly preach the Gospel. The baptism of the Holy Spirit empowers the believer to be a more effective witness. The gift of speaking in tongues is an empowerment and a tremendous tool in the context of deliverance. It can be evidence that a believer has experienced the baptism of the Holy Spirit, just as it was one sign of this experience on the Day of Pentecost; however, the primary evidence even on the Day of Pentecost was the empowerment of the disciples. The gift of tongues should not be overemphasized, as Scripture is equally clear that this is not the only sign of having been filled with the Holy Spirit. Prophecy is also a sign of this experience.

> *And when Paul had laid hands on them, the Holy Spirit came upon them, and they spoke with tongues and prophesied.*
> —*Acts 19:6* NKJV

Many nonbelievers who came into contact with the disciples became empowered believers whose lives were visibly changed. We know that the change in these believer's lives had some visible manifestation because "when Simon saw that through the laying on of the apostles' hands the Holy Spirit was given, he offered them money."[35]

The key phrase here is "when Simon saw." Simon saw a change in the lives of these believers—evidence that an impartation had occurred and that they had received the power.

Evidence of the Holy Spirit's Empowerment

The English word *empowerment* conveys the idea of an installation of power, especially legal power or official authority, and can also mean "to equip or to supply with an ability; to enable."[36] Empowerment is essential for successful deliverance ministry; however, it is merely the starting point for the installation of the authority that is also needed.

Official authority is conveyed to the believer in Luke 10:19, when Jesus states, "Behold, I give you the authority." The Holy Spirit teaches us and reminds us of the authority Jesus promised in Luke 10:19 and, according to Acts 1:8, has come that we might have power to be witnesses. So, just what does it mean to be a witness? The answer can be found in Mark 16.

And He said to them, "Go into all the world and preach the gospel to every creature. He who believes and is baptized will be saved; but he who does not believe will be condemned. And these signs will follow those who believe: In My name they will cast out demons; they will speak with new tongues; they will take up serpents; and if they drink anything deadly, it will by no means hurt them; they will lay hands on the sick, and they will recover."

—Mark 16:15–18 NKJV

One of the evidences of Holy Spirit empowerment is the ability to *look like* Jesus in the earth (in other words, to bear witness of Him), but it is the next step—walking in authority—that will enable us to begin to *act like* Jesus in the earth. As we are empowered by the Holy Spirit and start looking like Jesus, we become vessels to hold the gifts that He gives, including but not limited to, the ability to cast out demons in Jesus' name.

Scripture maintains that the Holy Spirit gives gifts to believers when He fills them. Among the gifts identified in 1 Corinthians 12 are several that have become essential in deliverance ministry. Two of the more prominent gifts used in deliverance are discerning of spirits and word of knowledge, which are mentioned in 1 Corinthians 12:8–10. The gift of discerning of spirits is helpful both in determining whether the problem is, at its core, demonic or carnal and whether the ministry recipient is speaking the truth. Words of knowledge can identify the root cause that allowed the enemy access in the first place and assist in closing that door.

Other gifts are also evidence of empowerment. The gift of healings can function side by side with casting out of demons, as has already been discussed. A word of wisdom can provide valuable insight as to when and how to proceed with ministry. The gift of faith, obviously, can have significant impact. If a person can say (without doubt), to the mountain, "Be removed," and it will be done,[37] then he or she can certainly say to demons, "Leave," and they will. Each of these gifts, in general or specifically in the context of deliverance ministry, shows the empowering role the Holy Spirit plays in our lives.

The Source of Authority

At first glance we might consider authority to be as much a gift as power is. Unfortunately, we all too often make this assumption, and as a result, we walk with very little authority at all. Consider Jesus' words.

> "It [the time when Jesus returns] is like a man going to a far country, who left his house and gave authority to his servants, and to each his work, and commanded the doorkeeper to watch."
>
> —Mark 13:34 NKJV

The question we must ask is, to whom did the man give his authority? The answer, of course, is that he gave it to his servants. The Greek word used here for servant is *doulos* (doo'-los), meaning a slave, but more specifically "one who gives himself up wholly to another's will and is devoted to another to the disregard of one's own interests."[38] Thus, it should be apparent that receiving authority is more than simply a gift; it also requires a close relationship with the Father—one in which we have set aside our own agenda in order to focus on His.

The parable used by Jesus in Mark 13 is about the Kingdom of God. The master who goes away is Jesus Himself, and the servants who received the master's authority were those who were "wholly devoted" to Him. Consider the closeness that Jesus had with the Father—He never said anything that the Father wasn't saying and never did anything that the Father wasn't doing.[39] This is the principle of slavery or servant-hood referred to in Mark 13—a lifestyle of absolute obedience. The evidence that a person has been given authority will ultimately be seen when then they exercise their God-given authority and produce fruit.

Romans 6:15–19 makes it clear that obedience is the key to establishing a deep relationship with God, thus resulting in authority. The implication is that we will present ourselves as slaves to something, either to sin or to obedience. By making ourselves the servants of obedience, the fruit produced in our lives will be righteousness and holiness, and the end result will be lives filled with authority.

The practice of building a deep relationship with the Father through obedience results in a lifestyle of holiness and righteousness. These qualities are developed in us when we become like little children and spend time with "Dad."

Using Kingdom authority changes everything, including the very way we attempt to demonstrate or display the Kingdom. When Jesus displayed Kingdom authority it changed the perception of ministry that existed in His day.

> But Jesus rebuked him, saying, "Be quiet, and come out of him!" And when the unclean spirit had convulsed him and cried out with a loud voice, he came out of him. Then they were all amazed, so that they questioned among themselves, saying, "What is this? What new doctrine is this? For with authority He commands even the unclean spirits, and they obey Him." And immediately His fame spread throughout all the region around Galilee.
> —Mark 1:25–28 NKJV (emphasis added)

We struggle to gather a group of people who love God together on a Sunday morning, but when Jesus displayed authority His fame spread and both the godly and the ungodly clamored to be near Him. Jesus walked in this kind of authority because He spent time with the Father. There was nothing in Him that was in common with the enemy He was confronting.[40]

Walking in true authority, as Jesus did, will not be taken lightly by our adversary. The source of real authority is found in righteousness and holiness. Authority is not based upon how much we know, but rather upon whom we know and how closely we know Him. To walk in real authority, it is not enough that we know about our Father, but rather we must truly know our Father, as Jesus knew Him. In this light, power must always precede authority (since it is the through the gift of the Holy Spirit that we are provided with the opportunity to know the Father as the Spirit knows Him), but the commitment to pursue the authority thereby offered must follow if we are to ever be truly successful in the ministry of deliverance.

Without question, every individual receives the Holy Spirit at the moment of salvation. The Word of God is clear that one cannot experience the wonder of salvation without the Holy Spirit's presence. However, Scripture is equally clear that the Holy Spirit's work doesn't stop there: He desires to empower all believers and to make them more effective witnesses of God. When believers accept the baptism of the Holy Spirit, their lives will be changed. There will be a visible difference that other believers and even nonbelievers will be able to see.

Individuals engaging in deliverance ministry would be wise to exert great care in choosing fellow ministry workers. Merely being a believer is not generally sufficient qualification for this ministry; being an empowered believer is preferable. However, God does honor our faith, and all believers (even without full, mature understanding of their power and authority) are ministers and can be used in unexpected ways and circumstances by God.

SECTION THREE
PRACTICAL SUGGESTIONS ON
DELIVERANCE

The first two sections of this book deal with foundational elements of deliverance ministry. Section Three offers practical suggestions for ministering to others: preparing a person to receive ministry, remaining free after ministry, and understanding limitations in ministry. Simply knowing one's enemy and oneself will enable an individual to minister to others, but these practical suggestions will make that ministry much easier and more effective. It is important that deliverance ministers not only understand the principles already discussed, but also know how to help others prepare for deliverance.

Remedy: Freedom Through Deliverance

CHAPTER 7

ENGAGING IN MINISTRY

People must be prepared to receive deliverance ministry, but the person ministering must also be ready for whatever could take place. Romans 12:10–12, though not specifically referring to deliverance ministry, serves as a code of conduct that deliverance ministers might take to heart.

> *Be kindly affectionate to one another with brotherly love, in honor giving preference to one another; not lagging in diligence, fervent in spirit, serving the Lord; rejoicing in hope, patient in tribulation, continuing steadfastly in prayer.*
> *—Romans 12:10–12 NKJV*

A sincere desire to see others set free can help overcome many of the difficulties associated with this ministry. The full strata of society are represented in the variety of those needing deliverance. The only thing they all have in common is that some open door in their life has allowed the enemy to gain a foothold. Quite frequently, this is uncomfortable for them to discuss, because habits of mind and/or body can be embarrassing or humiliating. A deliverance minister must maintain a tactful and compassionate, yet intrepid approach to the ministry recipients, even though the minister will frequently be confronted with issues that would cause many believers to want to run and hide rather than stand and fight. Only unconditional love can enable the minister to overcome such obstacles.

In addition, the deliverance minister must be willing to give preference to those in need of ministry. Giving preference doesn't mean the minister should bow down to every demand; rather, it means not allowing the minister's own preconceived notions of a person's character to cause a presumptuous judgment about the degree of deliverance that person needs. When we put others first, we place their needs ahead of our own and don't allow the desire for recognition on our part to interfere with what God is doing. Otherwise, we may assume others need deliverance merely because their personality type differs from or conflicts with our own, or because their life habits have created strongholds that need to be overcome. Through unconditional love and preferring others, the deliverance minister will also ensure that the proper time is taken to prepare the recipient to receive, instead of demanding he or she simply accept what the minister intends to do.

"Not lagging in diligence, fervent in spirit, serving the Lord"[41] are among the most challenging elements of this code of conduct. Just because the minister understands his or her own authority, power, and weapons does not ensure that every case will be an open-and-shut matter. The bottom line is that this service may require one to stand steadfastly and, having done all, simply to continue to stand.[42] It would be wonderful if we walked in the fullness of our authority in the same fashion that Jesus did, but it seems that most of us do not yet fully measure up to that standard.[43] When Jesus spoke, the work was done, but in our case, there will be times when we must persevere. In Acts 16, even Paul waited several days before finally ministering to the damsel with the spirit of divination, and when he did, the demon came out "that very hour,"[44] not necessarily meaning immediately.

It takes commitment to continue searching for the open door, teaching the person about deliverance, encouraging the person to forgive, and persisting in reaching them, even if the circumstances seem to offer no hope for success. Deliverance ministers must persevere, even in the face of rejection, for not everyone who needs this ministry accepts it with open arms; in fact, the deliverance minister can at times face open hostility.

Also, deliverance ministers must remember that a lack of immediate results does not equal failure. God's Word has always provided hope for the hopeless, and the trials and tribulations of deliverance ministry are merely the testing ground to mature everyone involved. Finally, those embarking on this ministry must be fully and absolutely committed to prayer, both as an element of preparation and as the primary weapon employed to set the captives free.

Demon Strongman versus Carnal Stronghold

Deliverance ministers must also discipline themselves to resist looking for a demon under every rock. One mistake made by those new to this ministry is attributing every problem to the demonic. In fact, both the deliverance minister and the recipient should begin *without* presuming deliverance is the answer. The need for deliverance should be suspected only after the normal channels of prayer, repentance, application of the Word, and other spiritual disciplines have been applied without a marked victory.

As already stated, the person receiving ministry must truly want to be free, no matter what way of life he or she has to give up or change. Sin is still sin and has consequences.

There is a clear difference between habitual sin that has established a carnal stronghold and an uncontrollable manifestation of a demonic strongman who has set up residence in or around the individual. When sin has reached the level where it is engaged in virtually without thought, it will open the door to demonic activity. But the individual's problem is not always a demon; it could be a stronghold.

A *stronghold* is defined as an area in an individual's life that has been surrendered to habitual sin. This can be a significant issue, since the minister has no authority over another individual's life. When a demon is the problem, the deliverance minister has absolute authority in Christ. But when the problem actually exists in the recipient's soul— that is, the mind, will, and emotions—a different approach is required. When the recipient's will is involved, the Holy Spirit will not violate that will, and He will not allow the minister to override it, either. Instead, the recipient must acknowledge the entrenched sin and be taught to overcome it.

When a person has clearly repented and taken the necessary steps to overcome his or her own carnal nature without success, we can then suspect demonic activity is operating. Too often, deliverance ministers feel they have failed because they have improperly tried to cast out the flesh, when the flesh should be disciplined, crucified, and overcome instead.

Teaching Those in Need to Aid in Their Own Deliverance

The deliverance minister must be a teacher, as well. (We are not suggesting that every believer will occupy the office of the teacher mentioned in Ephesians 4. We are simply pointing out that every believer has a responsibility to communicate the basic elements of the Gospel and that there is scriptural support for freedom from demonic harassment.) God's Word anticipates that those who come to Christ will share what they have learned with those around them. This expectation is no different for deliverance ministry. The person offering prayer and ministry has an understanding of how the demonic realm operates and how to travel the road to freedom that the person in need does not. Never overlook the importance of conveying this information as a prelude to actual ministry. The following seven points may seem foundational to the deliverance minister, yet they may be overlooked entirely by the one in need.

1. *Hate sin.* To be set free from demonic oppression, individuals must truly learn to hate sin. When we are born again, we acquire an aversion to sin via our God-given conscience, but we must also learn to actively repudiate sin, no matter how inconsequential it may seem.

2. *Desire complete freedom.* All too often, people seeking deliverance ministry desire to be set free from a specific problem, but not to be *free indeed.* Expressed another way, many people want to be free only from the problems caused by the demonic oppression, while hanging on to the potential benefits. To truly obtain total freedom, one must sincerely desire complete deliverance from all demonic activity. First Corinthians 5:6–7 uses the analogy of leaven in a loaf of bread. To paraphrase this verse, one could say that without complete freedom from demonic attack, everything just comes back.

3. *Reject the demonic.* Another common misconception among those seeking help is that they cannot get free by calling on God themselves. Taking authority as a believer and rejecting and renouncing the sin in one's own life are some of the first steps toward freedom. In some cases, this is all that is necessary. Even when prayer and ministry are needed, self-examination, evaluation, and subsequent action are fundamental. Remember, God's Word doesn't give authority only to pastors, evangelists, leaders, and those who minister deliverance, but it also gives authority to *you.* Every believer has access to the authority in Christ to subdue the enemy. At the very least, those in need of

deliverance should be taught the principle of binding and loosing found in Matthew 18:18.

4. *Get rid of reminders.* It is important for those who have been involved in overt demonic activity to rid themselves and their surroundings of any reminder of that involvement. While this may be taken to an extreme (such as believing no Christian should have any object shaped like a frog, resembling a frog, or depicting a frog), it is better to take this removal to an extreme than to ignore it altogether. All objects used in occult practices or sinful activity should be eliminated. Scripture confirms that such objects can be the focal point for demonic attack (see Acts 19:19, where many who had practiced magic brought their books together and burned them), and the enemy loves using these things to sow doubts about an individual's ability to overcome a particular sinful pattern.

5. *Prayer and fasting.* Anyone coming for ministry should understand the biblical principles of prayer and fasting and their accompanying power. An individual's preparation to receive ministry should be covered in prayer and instruction in the power incurred by fasting—a power that can multiply exponentially. When we exercise our will and overcome our flesh by denying it, we establish within ourselves a firm foundation for ministry. Self-denial through fasting demands that we elevate God's Word over our own desires and allow our spirit to take its rightful position of authority over our soul and flesh. Jesus Himself advised that some demonic spirits come out only through prayer and fasting.[45] Prayer as communication with the Holy Spirit enables both the deliverance minister and the recipient to share with the Father their concerns, desires, and questions in anticipation of His responses. Fasting prepares us to hear God's voice more accurately during ministry, and so, to be better prepared to give and receive.

As a side note, during ministry, ministry recipients should receive. It is not the time to engage actively in prayer, but time to allow the Holy Spirit to minister to them through the other believers present.

6. *Honesty.* For deliverance ministry to be successful, recipients should be encouraged to be completely honest and to hold nothing back, and ministers must be prepared for whatever they may hear. It is not required, nor in most cases even desirable, for recipients to share every detail of their lives. The Lord already knows these details.[46] Nevertheless, those undergoing deliverance must be willing to acknowledge the sin that has allowed the enemy's onslaught so that they can find freedom. Often, one of the enemy's most successful tactics is to convince us that the sin we hide cannot hurt us. In truth, hiding sin empowers it against us. Never forget who our enemy is and what his tools are. He is a master of deception and is not to be believed. The very nature of this ministry requires that we support a person's openness and honesty, but at the same time, we need to be wary of his or her truthfulness during the course of ministry itself. Since demons can and do speak through people, we must discern whether we are listening to the enemy or to the individual receiving ministry.

The following example shows how the enemy tries to deceive. On this occasion, the demonic entity stated that it wouldn't leave and that Bill had no authority to make it leave. Bill firmly told it that the Word of God gave him authority over demons, so it had to leave. At this point, in a high-pitched voice, Bill was told, "I'm gone." Unfortunately, this was not true, as was discerned both spiritually by the ministry team and physically by the nature of the statement itself. (Had the demon truly been gone, the individual would have said, "It's gone," instead of saying, "I'm gone.") After some additional ministry, the demonic entity left, and the individual was truly set free. This may seem humorous on the surface; however, it clearly illustrates that no matter how much you expect an individual to be honest with you, not every word uttered during a session can be trusted as truth.

7. *Physical manifestations/reactions.* Both those needing ministry and those ministering should be prepared for physical manifestations and/or reactions during the course of ministry. The Greek word for spirit is *pneuma* (pnyoo'-mah), which means "breath," and many demonic spirits are expelled in a breathy manner, such as through coughing, burping, sighing, yawning, screaming, weeping, vomiting, etc. Neither the recipient nor those ministering should be surprised or embarrassed by these manifestations. There could be other physical reactions, as well, but these should not cause undue alarm, either. It's also possible that successful deliverance ministry won't have any physical reaction whatsoever.

Conclusion

Engaging in deliverance ministry can be challenging and demanding. It requires a greater level of preparation than those receiving ministry. The deliverance minister's code of conduct is vital in this preparation. By focusing on God's Word, we can more easily overcome the enemy's attempts to distract us with negative manifestations.

Regarding demonic attempts to stop or at least frustrate deliverance ministry, it would appear the forces of darkness have taken to heart the familiar saying, "If you can't beat them, join them." Because of the natural tendency of someone new to this ministry to think demons are the cause of every difficulty, the enemy has successfully burned out many anointed ministers. By encouraging deliverance ministers to see a demon under every rock, the enemy attempts to overwhelm them and cause them to "grow weary in well-doing."[47]

Finally, the importance of teaching ministry recipients cannot be emphasized enough. They must have a basic understanding of what is about to take place and a familiarity with God's Word. The steps identified in this chapter help us prepare to engage in effective ministry and avoid any overconfidence in our own strength, which leads to failure.

Remedy: Freedom Through Deliverance

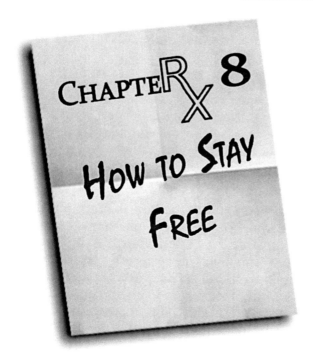

CHAPTER 8

HOW TO STAY FREE

Merely delivering an individual from demonic oppression is not enough. For deliverance ministry to be truly successful, ministers must also ensure that the recipient understands what it takes to remain free. This is why deliverance ministry is not recommended for unbelievers. For those receiving ministry, keeping their deliverance is as important as getting it—perhaps even more important. Jesus Himself explained the damage involved when a person does not maintain deliverance.

> "When an unclean spirit goes out of a man, he goes through dry places, seeking rest; and finding none, he says, 'I will return to my house from which I came.' And when he comes, he finds it swept and put in order. Then he goes and takes with him seven other spirits more

> *wicked than himself, and they enter and dwell
> there; and the last state of that man is worse
> than the first."*
>
> *—Luke 11:24–26* NKJV

Indisputably, if deliverance is not maintained, the situation becomes worse than before. Unclean spirits, or demons, are not content to leave on command and never return. Instead, while they may obey the believer's command, they remain ready and anxious to return to their former abode and continue their destructive work.

Teaching ministry recipients how to maintain their freedom is not optional. Deliverance ministers cannot afford to bypass this training. Such training is, however, quite difficult for unsaved people to use. If people don't comprehend even the basic principles of salvation, they probably will not understand the spiritual disciplines they must follow to maintain their freedom and not be able to apply them. In fact, when control of one's life has not been transferred from the god of this world to the God of the universe, a demonic oppressor's return is extremely likely.

How does a person maintain freedom after deliverance? By obeying God's Word. The following list of biblical life principles is far from exhaustive and should be practiced by every person who has received deliverance.

Yield every area of your life to the Lordship of Christ. This is a basic element of every Christian's life, yet it is surprising how many people do not understand it. Salvation recognizes Christ as Savior, but it is much more difficult for us to recognize Him as Lord. Believing on His name for salvation does not mean we're also bowing to His Lordship. Jesus warns us about those who call Him Lord but do not know Him as such.

> *"Not everyone who says to Me, 'Lord, Lord,' shall
> enter the kingdom of heaven, but he who does
> the will of My Father in heaven. Many will say
> to Me in that day, 'Lord, Lord, have we not*

prophesied in Your name, cast out demons in Your name, and done many wonders in Your name?' And then I will declare to them, 'I never knew you; depart from Me, you who practice lawlessness!'"
—*Matthew 7:21–23* NKJV

To be completely and consistently free from demonic oppression, one must yield control to Christ. Yielding complete control of one's life is not easy; nevertheless, we must strive to walk in this daily surrender. Also, we must confess immediately when we fail. First John 1:9 affirms that when we confess our sins, He is faithful and just to forgive us and to cleanse us from all unrighteousness.

Be continuously filled with the Holy Spirit. The Holy Spirit is the source of believers' power, and when we continually seek His infilling, we are strengthened. According to Paul, when we daily put to death the deeds of the flesh and are led by the Spirit, we have life.[48] The devil's role is to steal, kill, and destroy.[49] When we put to death the works of our flesh and live by the Spirit, we do not permit theft, death, or destruction to abide in us.

Live by the Word of God. Living by God's Word doesn't mean we simply believe it's true; it means we put it into practice. Jesus exemplified living by God's Word when Satan tempted Him in the wilderness. Jesus was tempted three times, and each time He responded, "It is written."[50] Jesus' statements were not merely a rote recitation of the memorized Word; they were life. They were the answer to the situation that He faced. He demonstrated to the enemy, and to us, that He not only knew God's Word but that He lived by it.

Put on the whole armor of God. The armor of God is our "uniform" of spiritual warfare, our "battle fatigues." This is true for both those ministering deliverance and those receiving and walking out their freedom. Ephesians 6:10–18 outlines the armor of God, which serves as protection and offensive positioning. The breastplate of righteousness and the shield of faith protect a soldier, while the sword of the Spirit can be an offensive weapon that reaches beyond the soldier's normal sphere of influence. However, donning the armor of God daily without walking in godly character is ineffectual. Wearing this armor entails more than merely confessing it as ours; it means living our lives in accordance with the characteristics of Christ. For example, it is not enough to say we are putting on the belt of truth; we must actually live our lives based on God's truth for the armor to operate effectively. These are weapons of the Spirit, and so, to bear these arms victoriously, one must walk in the Spirit.

Cultivate a renewed mind. Those who wish to live according to the Spirit set their minds on the things of the Spirit because being carnally minded brings death.[51] Paul tells us not to be conformed to the image of this world but transformed by the renewing of our minds.[52] The renewal of our mind is not a onetime prayer or deliverance, but a daily effort to fix our mind on godly, not worldly, pursuits.

Pray in the Spirit. Paul states that when one prays in a tongue, it is his or her spirit that prays,[53] and it speaks not to humanity but to God.

> *For he who speaks in a tongue does not speak*
> *to men but to God, for no one understands him;*
> *however, in the spirit he speaks mysteries.*
> —*1 Corinthians 14:2* NKJV

Also, according to 1 Corinthians 2:10, it is the Holy Spirit who searches out the deep things, who brings understanding to the mysteries spoken when one prays in tongues. Praying in tongues enables us to speak mysteries, not only confusing the enemy, but empowering us to pray effectively even when we don't know what to pray. It also edifies the one praying, strengthening his or her faith.[54] This increased ability to pray, to confuse the enemy, and to strengthen our faith makes tongues powerful ammunition for our lives and ministry.

Practice praise. Hebrews 13:15 admonishes us to continually offer our sacrifice of praise—the fruit of our lips—to God. This admonition means more than just being thankful, for thanksgiving is actually both offensive and defensive warfare against the demonic army. The offensive nature of praise is exemplified in the story of Jehoshaphat.[55] On the defensive side, praise is compared to one of the most significant defensive structures of biblical times: the gates of a city. God will be the defender; the gates of the city will experience no destruction and the sound of violence is not heard.[56]

Cultivate the right relationships. Right, loving relationships with our family in Christ create a strong foundation on which we can walk without stumbling.[57] In addition, 1 John 1:7 indicates that the blood of Jesus cleanses us from our sin as we walk in harmony with one another. Matthew 18:18–20 records Jesus' outline on maintaining proper relationships and ties this issue to several of the weapons used in deliverance (specifically the principles of binding and loosing and of agreement).

Develop a dynamic faith. Just as a lack of faith can be the basis for failure[58] and worries,[59] the presence of faith can be the source of victory.[60] To develop a dynamic faith, we must be cognizant about where we focus our attention. Both Mark and Luke record Christ's admonition to be careful of what we hear, because to those who hear, more will be given.[61] The importance of guarding our ears is further underscored when we recognize that faith comes by hearing and hearing by the Word of God.[62]

Practice confessing God's Word. Not only do we need to heed God's Word to develop a strong and dynamic faith, but we also need to know His Word to the extent that it becomes a part of us and flows out from us. To speak God's Word is to speak truth,[63] and truth will always defeat the enemy's plans. Jesus taught, "You shall know the truth, and the truth shall make you free."[64] By verbally confessing God's Word, we are both hearing the Word, which builds faith, and hiding it in our hearts. Luke 6:45 reminds us that out of the abundance of the heart, the mouth speaks.

Learn to crucify the flesh and resist the devil. Remember that our adversary, the devil, desires to drag those who have been set free back into the same bondage. The flesh is a battleground, and it must be put to death daily. God's Word exhorts us to crucify our old self and reckon ourselves dead to sin.[65] Paul conveys the struggle between flesh and spirit when he wrote that the things he desired to do he did not do, and the very things he desired not to do he did.[66] The battle is constant, but as we learn to crucify the flesh, we also learn to withstand the enemy's temptations and attacks. James reminds us that when we resist the devil, he will flee from us.[67] Our adversary may walk around as a roaring lion seeking to devour us, but if we remain steadfast and vigilant, we can overcome him.[68]

Avoid people who are a bad influence. God's Word firmly maintains that friendship with the world is enmity with God.[69] Numerous scriptures instruct us not to associate with the people whose influence may corrupt us. For example, Proverbs 22:24 advises us to not hang out with angry people. This doesn't mean we should avoid or reject unbelievers; after all, Jesus ministered to heathens and tax collectors—the untouchables of His culture. However, when we are trying to overcome the enemy and maintain our own personal freedom, it is wise not to comingle with people who will influence us to walk in bondage again.

Submit to the Lord and those in authority. Submission is not synonymous with obedience, both of which must be maintained if we are to keep our freedom. Submission connotes *willing obedience.* For example, a child who is told to sit down may obey but still not submit. He or she may sit down on the outside but *remain standing* on the inside. To maintain freedom, we must sit down both on the outside and on the inside. We cannot resist the enemy if we are not fully submitted to God. We should also humble ourselves and submit to those in authority so God can exalt us in His time.[70]

Maintain a daily prayer life. The Lord's Prayer demonstrates that we are to ask our Father to deliver us from the evil one.[71] This same passage also tells us how regular our prayer life needs to be: "Give us this day our daily bread."[72] Prayer is part of our spiritual sustenance, or bread, and it is to be part of our daily life.

Use your God-given weapons. Ephesians 6:17–18 identifies two of the offensive weapons in our arsenal: the sword of the Spirit (God's Word) and prayer. The principles of binding, loosing, and agreement are also offensive weapons, as well as the application of Jesus' blood to our circumstances and the use of His Name and authority.

Maintain a disciplined life. Paul stated that he disciplined his body and brought it into subjection so he would not be disqualified.[73] To maintain our freedom we, too, must live disciplined lives. We must recognize that living our lives for the Lord has clear rewards and offers present victory, but God's Word never promises that it is an easy road. On the contrary, we are warned that the gate is narrow, the way is difficult, and few find it.[74]

Fast regularly to keep the cutting edge in your life. Jesus taught that fasting was one part of the disciplined Christian life. He also taught that fasting should not be done for others to recognize and see but in secret, so the Father can reward us openly.[75] Fasting is a practice of self-denial to honor the Lord. By practicing fasting, we are acknowledging our commitment to keep the Father and His will as our center. By pursuing this type of close relationship with Him, we are effectively averting and defeating the enemy's snares and traps.

The points identified in this chapter are by no means a conclusive list of every action that should be taken to maintain a believer's freedom, but they are a biblically based foundation upon which to build. These foundational principles should be considered the minimum standard imparted to anyone who would receive deliverance ministry.

Those who minister in any area, but particularly in deliverance, should consider themselves watchmen set upon the wall. If the warning is given and the people ignore it, then their blood is upon themselves. Those who minister deliverance should warn (or teach) recipients what is required to maintain their freedom. If ministers fail to do so, the Lord may hold them responsible for any resulting damage.

> *But if the watchman sees the sword coming and does not blow the trumpet, and the people are not warned, and the sword comes and takes any person from among them, he is taken away in his iniquity; but his blood I will require at the watchman's hand.*
>
> —Ezekiel 33:6 NKJV

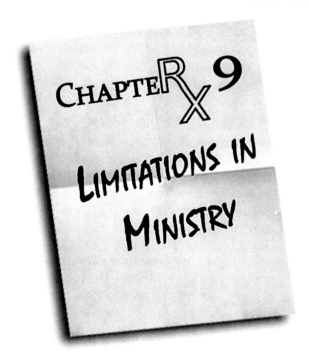

CHAPTER 9

LIMITATIONS IN MINISTRY

One of the greatest dangers for novice deliverance ministers is that they will exceed the authority granted them by God's Word or respond in such a way that excludes them from access to that authority in the first place. Deliverance is an act of warfare, and warfare is military action. God's Word clearly indicates that He considers us soldiers in virtually every area of our lives. Paul not only compared a believer to a soldier, but he also quite specifically and directly called the believer a soldier.

> *You therefore must endure hardship as a good soldier of Jesus Christ. No one engaged in warfare entangles himself with the affairs of this life, that he may please him who enlisted him as a soldier.*
>
> —*2 Timothy 2:3–4* NKJV

Recognizing that we are soldiers, we become aware of the danger of entangling ourselves with worldly affairs. Instead of allowing *civilian* matters to distract us, we must strive to act properly and under the command of the One who enlisted us—Jesus Christ. As good soldiers, we are expected not only to fight the good fight of faith,[76] but to follow the orders of Jesus, our Commanding Officer.

Believers have almost forgotten that army protocol is governed by rules of engagement, and these rules are provided to ensure both soldiers' and civilians' safety. Spiritual military life has its own rules of engagement so our army can be effective without causing collateral damage. Rules of engagement are typically codified and provided to each soldier so that he or she may know in advance how to handle a given situation. Just as with the natural structure of the military, God has His spiritual army, and we are expected to obey His written and oral directives.

God's rules of engagement are our guidelines for spiritual warfare. They inform us when to refrain from battle and when to press in. They train us for guerilla warfare and sabotage. The following points are some fundamental areas in which believers should exercise caution when ministering deliverance or engaging in spiritual warfare. If unsuccessful in deliverance ministry, these are some of the first issues to examine.

Violation of an Individual's Will

God created humans to have a degree of free will. How far that free will extends may be debatable, but its existence is unquestionable. In the Garden of Eden, humanity chose to exercise that free will and believe a serpent's lies over God's truth. As a result, sin entered the world and humanity's relationship with God was broken. This broken relationship allows Satan's demonic forces to harass, intimidate, and oppress or possess humankind.

Whenever we attempt to unseat a demonic entity from its throne of influence over a person, place, or thing, a battle must be waged. As we discussed earlier, both Christians and non-Christians can consent to evil influences in their lives. As a result, one of the first hurdles to overcome in deliverance ministry is to ensure that the recipient actually wants to be free. This may seem to be a rather juvenile concern until we recognize how the enemy employs his primary weapon of deception.

The serpent's tactics were lies from the beginning. In the Garden, he convinced Eve that God's motives were questionable and she had nothing to lose and everything to gain by eating from the Tree of the Knowledge of Good and Evil. Since the enemy operates within the framework of deception, it should not be surprising that some individuals may be deceived into believing nothing is wrong and they are perfectly fine just the way they are.

Deliverance will not benefit an individual who does not want to be free. Demons have no authority in a believer's life except what the believer gives them. To seek individuals' freedom from influences that will immediately be allowed to return is of no benefit whatsoever. Deliverance should never be ministered in a context where the individual has not purposefully expressed a desire to be free from demonic influence (either generally or specifically).

Evil spirits do not simply leave when commanded to do so and never return. Quite the contrary, when they are driven out, they actively seek to return...with comrades. For unbelievers, this will result in worse bondage than before. Jesus referred to deliverance (and healing) as the "children's bread" because of this reason. It is unlikely unbelievers will understand how to avert the demonic entity's return, particularly when they do not have Christ to lean on for continued freedom.

When the unclean spirit seeks to return to its former home, it is able to because those quarters are unoccupied. By extension, it would appear that in order to avoid the demon's return (along with seven additional wicked spirits), the house must be occupied with something else.

> *"When an unclean spirit goes out of a man, he goes through dry places, seeking rest; and finding none, he says, 'I will return to my house from which I came.' And when he comes, he finds it swept and put in order. Then he goes and takes with him seven other spirits more wicked than himself, and they enter and dwell there; and the last state of that man is worse than the first."*
>
> —Luke 11:24–26 NKJV

The first step in occupation is for the believer to turn over dominion of that area of his or her life to the Holy Spirit. The next step is to allow the Holy Spirit to fill his or her life with love, joy, peace, and all the other fruits of the Spirit. Obviously, these are acts requiring decisions of the will. So, unwanted or nonconsensual deliverance often creates more problems than it solves and ultimately does more harm than good. But how can unwanted or nonconsensual deliverance even occur? If those ministering deliverance choose to exercise their authority over demons without the recipient having a true desire to be free, then he or she will make no effort to fill that empty space with the fruit and presence of the Holy Spirit and may overtly, or even subtly, welcome the demonic presence back into his or her life. And as Scripture attests, the latter state of that person will be worse than the first.

Two factors are at work here. First, believers have access to the authority to command demons to leave but not to ensure that they do not return. (That is the responsibility of the person receiving ministry.) Second, demons clearly know and understand God's Word and its principles (recall that Satan twisted God's Word to deceive Eve in the

Garden[77] and to tempt Jesus in the wilderness[78]), so they may willingly depart until an opportune time to return in greater numbers.

Some people have attempted to ignore this issue of the misuse of deliverance ministry and, in one sense, use deliverance as a tool to "fix" a person in hopes that they will come to Christ or in response to some sort of crisis. Frequently those who use deliverance in this way will justify their actions on the basis of sending the demonic entities to the abyss or commanding them never to return. Unfortunately, there is little biblical support for such an action. While the demons who identified themselves as "Legion" begged to not be sent into the abyss, they also begged for Jesus to not torment them.[79] Notice that Jesus did not send them away into the abyss. Revelation 20 indicates that there is a specific time at which Satan will be bound and even then loosed for a little while after a thousand years in order to entice the earth again. By extrapolation, this would seem to indicate that Satan and his demonic forces have a set time that they are free to operate in the earth and it would seem that it cannot be changed by our command. Certainly we cannot control whether or not a person will "allow" the demonic to return. With these precepts in mind, it is best to use wisdom and never act in ways that would violate the will of an individual who is not ready to be free, and instead focus our attention on seeking to reveal the truth of God's Word to them in a fashion that would create a hunger for freedom.

Lack of Preparation

Jesus is our role model. He discipled others in the works He performed, demonstrated His authority to them, and sent them out two by two with power to heal and deliver. With this level of preparation and instruction, the disciples were successful at casting out demons and healing people.[80] One of the main reasons for failure in ministering deliverance is the lack of preparation before stepping out into action. The disciples exercised great authority, nevertheless there came a time when they were unsuccessful in their deliverance ministry.

Mark 9:17–29 describes a situation when the disciples had had an opportunity to cast out a spirit but were unsuccessful. Jesus, on the other hand, spoke and it was accomplished. When the disciples questioned Jesus privately about why they had been unsuccessful, He basically told them it was due to their unpreparedness.

> *And when He had come into the house, His disciples asked Him privately, "Why could we not cast it out?" So He said to them, "This kind can come out by nothing but prayer and fasting."*
> —Mark 9:28–29 NKJV

Jesus' statement, "This kind can come out by nothing but prayer and fasting," reveals much more than just information on how to exorcise a specific type of demonic spirit. Jesus showed the disciples that they had become complacent. The disciples presumed Jesus' authority was sufficient, when in reality, their own preparation for warfare was also important. The preparation they lacked involved receiving marching orders and carrying those orders out. First, they had not spent the time necessary in prayer to know from God how to handle this specific situation. Second, they had not exercised self-discipline (fasting) to prepare themselves to accomplish the work.

The Lord is merciful and often honors our efforts even when our preparation has been lacking; and yet, He expects to see a continual maturing process in us. We must graduate from milk to meat at a certain stage. There is a price to be paid in deliverance ministry if we enter a situation without proper preparation. When we find ourselves in an unforeseen spiritual battle, God will certainly uphold us; however, when we know we will face spiritual warfare, it is important to be adequately prepared so we can achieve victory easily and swiftly, with minimal casualties and damage.

Using Our Own Knowledge

Lack of preparation can lead to serious faults in deliverance ministry. One of the most serious is ministering out of our own knowledge rather than God's revelation. When we fail to prepare, we will often fail to listen to what God is saying and look for what He is doing. God is not comprehended by our intellect; even the demons believe in God and tremble.[81]

Tools such as lists of demonic strongholds, checklists to identify a person's sinful activities, written or memorized prayers, etc., can be beneficial in deliverance ministry, but it is also important to let God orchestrate each unique situation. Formulas and methodologies based on human knowledge may be useful as reminders, but they can never substitute for God's direction, for all can potentially fail, but God will not. One of the most famous biblical examples of following a format without divine input occurs in Acts.

> Then some of the itinerant Jewish exorcists took it upon themselves to call the name of the Lord Jesus over those who had evil spirits, saying, "We exorcise you by the Jesus whom Paul preaches." Also there were seven sons of Sceva, a Jewish chief priest, who did so. And the evil spirit answered and said, "Jesus I know, and Paul I know; but who are you?" Then the man in whom the evil spirit was leaped on them, overpowered them, and prevailed against them, so that they fled out of that house naked and wounded.
>
> —Acts 19:13–16 NKJV

The lesson here is that invoking the name of Jesus held sufficient authority to cast out demonic powers—but not without dialogue and relationship with Jesus. Notice that when the seven sons of Sceva acted on information rather than revelation or communication with God, the enemy (or the demonic spirit) prevailed. Acting on presumption without relationship and revelation can seriously injure us, but when we walk in the fullness of the power and authority God has granted us, nothing can harm us.[82]

Divine revelation provides breakthroughs in challenging deliverance situations. Once while ministering to a woman who had been a high priestess in satanism, Bill and his ministry team had reached a dead end. However, during an afternoon walk in the woods, the Lord spoke to one of Bill's team members and told him to pull a flower from a dogwood tree. The Lord then identified four remaining demonic entities and using the crown (pistil and stamen) in the middle of the flower, He identified a fifth demon that remained, which was recognized as the strongman in this woman's life. This revelation was the breakthrough needed to exorcise those demonic spirits. Applying human knowledge without divine revelation in such a situation would have severely hampered the effort to set this woman free.

Reviling the Enemy

An easy mistake in deliverance ministry is to be drawn into arguments with demonic entities. Demons often speak through individuals. It is important to distinguish throughout the deliverance session between the voice of the ministry recipient and the voices of the demonic entities speaking through him or her. Arguments with demons often begin with a simple exchange:

> Minister: "I command you to go in the name of Jesus."
> Demon: "I won't leave."
> Minister: "You have to leave."
> Demon: "I do not."
> Minister: "Yes, you do."
> Demon: "I won't go."
> Minister: "You must go."

It is not unusual for inexperienced deliverance ministers to begin with a similar dialogue and before they've realized it, to be arguing rather than ministering. Such a situation is designed by the enemy to misdirect the interaction, create distraction, and belie the truth of God's Word and the believer's authority. By doing this, the enemy succeeds in drawing attention away from Jesus and the authority of His name and redirects the focus on the demonic entity and its will. Satanic forces seize every opportunity to lie, provoke, and intimidate in order to maintain their positions.

Once an argument is initiated by a demon, the minister then risks having it become an interchange of a reviling nature. A reviling conversation occurs when the exchange shifts to verbal abuse, scolding, quarreling, or angry rebukes. The minister at that point has been lured into the enemy's trap. The key scriptural admonition against this pitfall is found in Jude.

> Yet Michael the archangel, in contending with the devil, when he disputed about the body of Moses, dared not bring against him a reviling accusation, but said, "The Lord rebuke you!"
> —Jude 9 NKJV

Refusing to engage in disparaging and scornful conversation keeps the focus of deliverance ministry on the authority of the Lord Jesus Christ. If the enemy can provoke the minister to agitation, anger, and frustration, then he can successfully thwart deliverance.

Exercising Celestial Authority

Human beings, in our fallen state, have forever sought to dominate and control whatever we can. Frequently, though, we have attempted to wield authority where we have no "legal" right to intervene. Deliverance ministry is no exception, and the results can be devastating. God's Word proclaims that in the beginning, humankind was given dominion over the earth.[83] However, nowhere in God's Word are we given dominion in the heavens or over other human beings. One of the strictest limitations in deliverance ministry (and in spiritual warfare in general) is the biblical limitation on the human realm of authority.

When we seek to exercise authority where God has not granted it, we move ourselves outside the protective covering of God's grace and make ourselves vulnerable to the enemy's counterattacks. It is vital to remember that the basis of our authority is God's Word. There is a price to be paid and needless casualties may ensue when we attempt to exercise authority we do not hold. God's Word delineates the boundaries of human authority.

The initial grant of human authority happened in the Garden of Eden when God gave Adam dominion over the earth and all its inhabitants. It was a limited grant of authority, or in legal terminology, a limited power of attorney. Adam and Eve's fall relinquished human dominion over the earth to Satan, a loss that could only be reversed through divine redemption. The finished work of Christ on the cross returned legal authority over the earth to God, and Jesus' sacrifice resulted in His exaltation, placing all authority in His hands.

Jesus said "all authority has been given to Me in heaven and on earth."[84] This statement clearly indicates at least two realms of authority: one in heaven and one on earth. As disciples of Jesus, our authority is to be exercised in an earthly, not heavenly, context. Jesus explains the relationship of our authority on earth and in heaven in Matthew 18.

> *"Assuredly, I say to you, whatever you bind on earth will be bound in heaven, and whatever you loose on earth will be loosed in heaven. Again I say to you that if two of you agree on earth concerning anything that they ask, it will be done for them by My Father in heaven."*
> —*Matthew 18:18–19* NKJV

The authority given to believers to trample serpents and scorpions (symbolic of demons and devils) is earthly authority. We have the legal right to tread them under our feet. This indicates believers' absolute, earthly authority over demonic activity and, therefore, authority to minister deliverance. We have this right because the demonic entity has stepped into our realm of authority. However, we would be exceeding our authority if we attempted to rebuke or command demonic forces that have not entered the earthly realm. More specifically, in deliverance, we always have authority to command demons oppressing individuals to depart; however, we do not have the authority to come against a ruling principality that is overseeing a demonic onslaught from its second heaven position (the demonic realm).

Daniel 10 is the basis for the understanding of earthly and heavenly realms.

> Suddenly, a hand touched me, which made me tremble on my knees and on the palms of my hands. And he said to me, "O Daniel, man greatly beloved, understand the words that I speak to you, and stand upright, for I have now been sent to you." While he was speaking this word to me, I stood trembling. Then he said to me, "Do not fear, Daniel, for from the first day that you set your heart to understand, and to humble yourself before your God, your words were heard; and I have come because of your words. But the prince of the kingdom of Persia withstood me twenty-one days; and behold, Michael, one of the chief princes, came to help me, for I had been left alone there with the kings of Persia. Now I have come to make you understand what will happen to your people in the latter days, for the vision refers to many days yet to come."...Then he said, "Do you know why I have come to you? And now I must return to fight with the prince of Persia; and when I have gone forth, indeed the prince of Greece will come. But I will tell you what is noted in the

> *Scripture of Truth. (No one upholds me against these, except Michael your prince."*
> —Daniel 10:10–14, 20–21 NKJV

In this story, we learn that Daniel's prayers had no effect upon the warfare taking place in the heavens. In fact, the answer to Daniel's prayer was delayed by that warfare. This angelic being who spoke to Daniel acknowledged that he had come because of Daniel's words, yet those same words had been unable to impact the twenty-one-day demonic opposition. Apparently, Daniel commanded authority in the earthly realm, but lacked it in the realm of the second heaven. When the angelic being left Daniel to return to the battle, he noted that "no one" was available to assist him except the angel Michael. No one else had the authority to do so. Despite Daniel's limited authority, this warfare did not stop the answer to his prayer, for God has authority even in the second heaven and can delegate it to whom He will (in this case, to the angel Michael and the angel who visited Daniel).

Since we presently exist within the confines of the earthly realm, our authority mirrors that of Daniel; just as Daniel's impact on the second heaven was limited, so are we limited in our spiritual warfare. Because we exist within the confines of the earthly realm, any demonic power that would oppress us must enter that realm and so becomes an open target of believers' spiritual warfare.

For detailed information on this limitation of spiritual warfare, we recommend the book *Needless Casualties of War* by John Paul Jackson.

The Issue of Defilement

The basis for deliverance ministry, in fact for all ministry, is that the believer might do the things that Jesus did and even greater things.[85] The idea that we could do anything that Jesus did is of course based upon the assumption that we would be striving to be like Him and that in becoming like Him we grow more mature, looking more and more like our Father with each passing day.[86] With this premise in mind, anything that might cause us to look less like our Father would by necessity limit our ability to do the things that Jesus did, including the casting out of demons. The light of God within each of us must shine in such a way that it penetrates the darkness caused by the presence of the evil one. In order for that light to properly shine, we must guard our hearts and minds that we might walk in the righteousness of God through Christ Jesus. Matthew 13:43 indicates that it is the righteousness of God that shines forth like the sun in the Kingdom of God. When that light so shines, the darkness of the demonic world has no hope of victory.

On the other hand, when the light of God within us is diminished, even to a small degree, then darkness may find a way to remain. It should, therefore, be our desire to allow the full brightness of the Son to shine through us in order to confound the works of the enemy around us. Anything that causes our thoughts or actions to become unclean will by necessity result in the light of God that we carry within us being less visible from us. This raises the issue of defilement as a limitation on the effectiveness of our ministry. Defilement can be defined as making something unclean, or sullying it. Thus when we are defiled, our lives become soiled or tarnished, and our light is diminished. If we desire to be effective in the ministry of deliverance, then we must take this matter seriously.

In the book of Mark, Jesus taught that it was those things that come out of us that defile us.[87]

When our hearts are filled with evil thoughts and ungodly desires, then we become defiled. The book of James goes on to identify that the manifestation of sin that shows up in our actions begins when the thoughts and desires within us conceive and give birth to it. The book of Galatians makes clear that those things will hinder our inheritance of the Kingdom of God.[88] Since deliverance from the demonic is a principle of the Kingdom of God, when we are defiled from within, our ability to release the manifestation of that principle is hindered. When we read passages such as Mark 7 and Galatians 5, we often have the tendency to think of such defilements as major sin issues in our life; however, when we more carefully examine these passages, we find the underlying language to encompass things that we often think of as less severe, such as: pride, foolishness, hostility, quarrelling, and the lack of unity. All of these and many other "innocent" thoughts and feelings can lead to defilement.

Certainly, we are covered by grace; however, we do have a responsibility to walk clean before the Lord. If we fall into the trap of obeying those thoughts and feelings that lead to defilement and sin, then we once again present ourselves as slaves to sin and thereby to Satan.[89] When we walk in defilement, we begin to have something in common with the very demonic world that we are seeking to confront. In speaking of His coming death, Jesus told the disciples that "the ruler of this world (Satan) had nothing in Him."[90] In other words, Jesus had nothing in common with the forces of darkness that He was confronting. The light of God within Him was not diminished and shone like the sun to drive the demonic out of those in need of freedom.

Consider the "minor" issues in our own lives and how they can then affect our ability to minister deliverance. If, for example, we have an issue with contention (quarrelling) or dissension (lack of unity), then we have something in common with those "minor" demonic powers, and our ability to command them to depart is hindered. This becomes even more problematic if we consider other New Testament principles, such as the fact that Jesus equated the sin of anger in our heart with the sin of murder.[91] We cannot expect to deal with the disobedience of the demonic until our obedience is fulfilled.

> *For the weapons of our warfare are not carnal*
> *but mighty in God for pulling down strongholds,*
> *casting down arguments and every high thing*

that exalts itself against the knowledge of God, bringing every thought into captivity to the obedience of Christ, and being ready to punish all disobedience when your obedience is fulfilled.

—2 Corinthians 10:4–6 NKJV

In order to fulfill our own obedience, we must deal with the issue of defilement by dealing with the very thoughts and intents of our heart and ensuring that we are a pure and clean vessel for the light of God to shine through.

Remedy: Freedom Through Deliverance

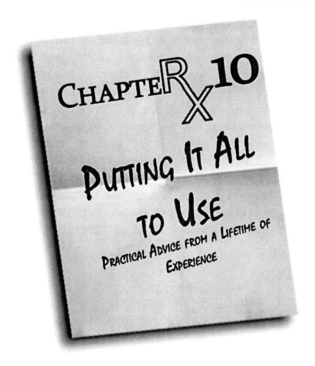

CHAPTER 10

PUTTING IT ALL TO USE

PRACTICAL ADVICE FROM A LIFETIME OF EXPERIENCE

For too long, deliverance was the subject of hushed conversations in the back rooms of the Church. A necessary component of spiritual life, the practical applications raised many questions and created messes that most of the Church didn't want to deal with. When Bill first began to move in this area of ministry, it was perhaps subject to more rejection within the Church than from without. Witchcraft, Wicca, voodoo, satanism, neo-paganism, and dozens of other occult/pagan religious systems were practiced only in secret, and on the heels of the "God is dead" argument; the devil and demons seemed of little concern. Today, with all of these belief systems vying for their place of prominence in popular culture and occult-related crime rampart on the nightly news, the reality of the demonic hits much closer to home.

Remedy: Freedom Through Deliverance

Even in the midst of such open occultism, the average believer will rarely encounter the need to minister to a true witch, druid, or warlock. Instead, everyday issues that result from demonic oppression are much more common. Unfortunately, it is some of these common issues that open the door to deeper involvement in the realm of the occult, and if left unchecked, can develop into major problems as they build up over time. With that in mind, it is the intention of this chapter to outline two or three seemingly innocuous issues that seem to give rise to the need for deliverance ministry on a somewhat consistent basis and to add some additional real-life experiences to help understand more of the practical application of deliverance ministry.

Common Issues

Trauma

It is not uncommon for the demonic to use a doorway of trauma to gain access to the life of an individual. In psychological terms, *trauma* is considered to be an emotional response to a terrible event such as an accident, an abusive incident, or involvement in or observation of a disaster of some sort. From a definitional standpoint, *trauma* is considered a serious injury or shock to the body or an emotional wound that has lasting impact upon a personal psychological condition. In a medical sense, *trauma* can also be defined in relationship to the physical responses of the body to severe injury.

In all of these cases, a doorway to demonic activity or influence can be opened in the life of the individual who has been subjected to trauma. It is difficult to discern exactly why this occurs, but it could be considered to be the result of a person being in a more fragile spiritual state when such trauma occurs. This is especially true when trauma occurs during childhood and can even have significant impact when trauma is experienced by a mother while a child is in the womb.

It is important to recognize that we cannot change the past. If trauma has occurred it cannot be undone; however, we can change the way we respond to it in the present and future. In order for deliverance to be effective where the doorway to the demonic has been opened through trauma, it is not necessary to undo what took place, but rather to recognize that it no longer has to continue to affect and/or impose direction in our lives. Often our responses to the traumatic events or circumstances begin quite naturally, but through fear, anxiety, or other common emotional responses, the enemy finds a way to exaggerate those responses to a point that they become detrimental and manipulative in our lives.

Imaginary Friends

For most people the idea of an imaginary, invisible friend would be limited to the carefree days of childhood. Some of those who read this book may have had imaginary friends as children, and others may have children who have them. As this topic is examined, it should be important to recognize that there are certainly occasions when the imaginary friend of a child is nothing more than that—a figment of a fanciful childhood imagination. However, there are also other possible explanations, including the presence of either angelic or demonic beings, and it is this possibility that raises the discussion in the context of a book on spiritual warfare and deliverance. Because both of these possibilities exist, it is often best for parents to initially address this matter through prayer and spiritual warfare, rather than confronting the matter head-on with the child at the outset.

The imaginary childhood friend, with which we are concerned, is not found in the setting of the preschool girl sitting at the table having a tea party with an imagined collection of children, dolls, and stuffed animals. Neither is it found in the setting of a small boy fighting alongside his imaginary company of warriors, knights, or soldiers against an unseen onslaught of enemy forces. These casual, yet vivid events are almost inevitably the product of healthy and normal childhood imagination and a playful heart.

It is important to recognize that western culture has all but dismissed that which exists in the unseen spiritual realm. Instead we favor the notion that only what we can see, hear, feel, taste, and touch could possibly be real. In so doing, we have also learned to train our children that what would otherwise be very real and valid spiritual experiences are nothing more than a product of their overactive imaginations. It is imperative that we begin to recognize that in too many cases, it is we—the adults—who have been deceived and that the world seen through the innocence of a child's eyes may actually be far bigger than we can any longer imagine. When a child sees into the spiritual world around them, depending on the environment in which they find themselves and the spiritual circumstances that they are confronted with, they may truly be seeing into a realm of either light or darkness. That large, strong man who helped to keep them safe and comforted them when they were afraid might very well be an angel. (After all, the Word of God is clear that we sometimes entertain angels unaware.[92]) On the other hand, that monster under the bed might very well be a demonic manifestation designed to terrify them and destroy their willingness to gaze into the spiritual realm as they mature. It is important to remember that such typical responses can also be reversed, as demonic entities can present themselves in a very pleasant manner at first and angels can certainly invoke a sense of reverential fear.

How parents handle situations such as these can have a significant impact upon whether or not a child continues to accept that they can hear and see on a spiritual level as they grow older. Too frequently, our culture has destroyed this sensitivity rather than supported it. Parents are quick to dismiss both the protector and the monster as an overactive imagination or an ill-conceived attempt to stay up a little later or to join mom and dad in their room.

Responses such as "there are no such things as monsters" and "that's sweet, but it wasn't real" reinforce the idea that only what we can discern with our natural senses is real. Having come this far in the reading of this book, it would be likely that you no longer accept this premise as truth (if in fact you ever did) and thus must reconsider the use of such dismissive responses as explanation for events that we have difficulty explaining.

Perhaps when faced with such circumstances, it would be better to explain the very real existence of a coexisting spiritual world and seek to understand what the child might be experiencing rather than dismissing it outright. To do so might result in avoiding the problem discussed in this chapter at the outset rather than having to deal with the demonic influence after it has already become an established issue in the child's life. Children are engaged in the warfare that exists in the spiritual world just as much as adults. By training our children that we have both spiritual enemies and spiritual allies, we can help them to understand the spiritual experiences that they are often far more prone to than we are. Calling upon angelic assistance and standing against the forces of darkness are principles that too many people learn too late in life.

The imaginary friend (or perhaps more appropriately the invisible friend) with which we are concerned is one that is invisible to everyone else, but quite real and even visible to the child with whom they interact. These "friends" are not filled with light and intent upon edifying, protecting, and encouraging the child, but rather dark and negative or neutral at best (though at times appearing friendly, sympathetic, and helpful—like the angel of light described in 2 Corinthians 11:14). They are demons in disguise. In most cases, such "friends" can be described down to the last detail: how they dress, what they look like, how they act, what they talk about, and even how the child gets them to show up. It is not uncommon for such "friends" to be described in such detail, yet never to have allowed their face to be seen. (For example, the friend is always wearing a mask or the friend never looks directly at the child.) Often, children who are experiencing these demonic manifestations will become upset or even angry when someone sits in the "friend's" seat or insists that the child leave before the "friend" is ready to go. Unfortunately, the cultural tendency to dismiss such protests and the failure to recognize that something spiritual might be at work can actually worsen the situation and drive the child into the confidence of the "demonic friend."

Demonic childhood "friends" frequently appear around the time a child turns two or three years old and are often gone by the time they reach the age of six or seven. The disappearance most often is only from the natural, visible realm and is typically a result of the child having been finally convinced that it was their imagination and that the "friend" doesn't actually exist. In other cases, the "friend" simply quits appearing because of a concern that the child may be growing old enough to actually discern what is really going on. In either case, the demonic entity doesn't give up and leave, but rather lingers and becomes an oppressive influence for the rest of the child's life unless it is dealt with as any other oppressive demonic entity would be. While the demonic "friend" may have acted quite benevolently while it was seen, as time passes the influence that it exerts becomes much more malevolent.

In some extreme cases, these imaginary "friends" never disappear and in others they may eventually be replaced by adult imaginary "friends" or family members. On at least one occasion, Bill ministered to an individual in her late forties who had an entire imaginary family, including a husband and three children. While there was absolutely no visible indication of this problem, the imaginary family was so real to the individual that she bought the children clothes and had parties for them. She had become so dependent on the imaginary family that she didn't want to be free or get rid of them. Cases such as these, of course, have every potential of resulting in what seems to be serious mental illness unless the person becomes willing to be set free.

Although a distinction between the vivid imagination of a young child and the demonic influence of a spiritually real imaginary friend has been made, it is important that this distinction be clearly understood. As has previously been emphasized, it is inappropriate to look for a demon as the cause of every issue that arises in a person's life, but when such influence does exist in the form of an imaginary friend it is essential that it not be overlooked. Simply put, the childhood imaginary friends with which we are concerned are demonic entities, whose ultimate goal is to bring emotional upheaval and instability in the life of the child or later in their adulthood. As the demonic foothold strengthens, the adult who has not received freedom from this demonic influence begins to see the upheaval in their life as natural and normal, because they have "always been that way."

Because of the age at which these demonic entities begin to manifest, it is often difficult to determine the exact cause or root of their appearance. The door to this influence can open as the result of loneliness, neglect, abuse/childhood trauma, generational curses, family activities, or any number of other possibilities. Regardless of the root issue, the principles expressed in the pages of this book can be applied to ensure that freedom comes from the darkness that has sought to consume these lives. If possible, an early intervention is beneficial due to the initial appearance of benevolence that such an imaginary friend uses in order to gain trust and hide its true nature.

Chemical Imbalance

Mental instabilities are sometimes referred to as chemical imbalances in the brain. Some of these cases are due to physical conditions, while others may be a result of outside influences such as drugs or alcohol. In either event, such cases usually involve behavioral or emotional patterns that are disruptive and/or out of order. For example, it is not at all uncommon for someone with a drug addiction to come to seek assistance from an individual or ministry team that understands deliverance ministry. Nor is it uncommon for a person suffering from a mental health issue to pursue deliverance as a possible course of relief.

It is important to recognize that while these may be common issues, deliverance is frequently not the sole solution for such concerns. Whether the imbalance results from a natural physical disorder or from an outside influence like substance abuse, there is likely to be both a spiritual and a physical issue that must be dealt with. Freedom from demonic oppression does not necessarily solve the problem in its entirety. On the other hand, hospitalization, recovery programs, and even physical healing may not provide the complete solution, either. In such cases, it is important to recognize that, if the part you play is that of one who ministers deliverance, it is essential that all of the other related needs be addressed, as well. This may mean praying for physical healing and a restoration of the physical functions of the body that had been influenced or disrupted by the demonic entity. It can also mean that additional counseling to help change habitual behavior or addictive tendencies can be helpful, and in some such cases, it may be appropriate for the individual to seek professional counseling assistance from a Christian perspective. Especially in the case of issues that can be described along the lines of a chemical imbalance in the brain, the deliverance minister should maintain the recognition that they serve as one part of a many-membered body[93] and that other parts may also be needed in order to see a person completely set free, healed, and restored.

The Night Season

The battle that we are engaged in is a battle between light and darkness. Perhaps everyone is familiar with the words of 1 John 4:8 that declares "God is love"; however, far fewer realize that prior to these words (in 1 John 1:5) the writer declares that "...God is light and in him is no darkness at all." With these words in mind, it would not be unusual to find that much of the warfare in which we are engaged takes place during the night season, when darkness covers the earth. It is in this night realm that the enemy finds his greatest opportunity to sow the seeds of fear, anxiety, and worry. The demonic world recognizes that there is a greater opportunity for destruction when they are cloaked in the darkness of night.

Consider for a moment the number of people who have difficulty sleeping soundly through the night. In the natural order of things, the night season should be our time of rest and refreshing, a time to renew our energy in order to face another day and move in the things that God has given us to do. The need for sleep in order to continue to function in a natural capacity will also have an impact upon our spiritual life, and it is perhaps also for this reason, that the enemy chooses to assault the minds and lives of those who he can in order to disrupt this cycle of rest. According to the psalmist this attack against the rest of a believer should not have to be endured.

> *I will both lie down in peace, and sleep; for You alone, O LORD, make me dwell in safety.*
> —*Psalm 4:8* NKJV

For those troubled by the demonic, both Christian and non-Christian alike, the peace that should come with sleep can be stolen, and the dwelling place of safety that sleep should provide can be lost. Difficulty going to sleep, awaking frequently through the night, having nightmares and bad dreams, all of which may have perfectly natural (non-spiritual) explanations, can also be an indication of demonic oppression. We should never become so obsessed with the enemy's role in causing a disruption in a night's sleep that we forget that God can also awaken us for prayer.

Many times, a difficulty with sleeping is related to the over-activity of the mind, as every possible idea and/or imagination begins to steamroll its way through the individual's thoughts. This traffic in the mind can be tormenting, and the turmoil it causes can paralyze the decision-making processes in addition to disrupting sleep patterns. For some, this prevents sleep from coming, and for others, it may awaken them through the night or early in the morning. Such disruption can also have a significant impact on the ability to function during the daylight hours, as well. This can be true even when it appears that there has been a sufficient amount of sleep due to the tremendous spiritual warfare that is taking place behind the scenes. While there are many natural causes for disrupting patterns such as these, there are also spiritual issues that can be at work. Guilt, unforgiveness, sinful patterns of behavior, inability to let go of the past, hidden issues, and more can all open the door to demonic influence during the night season.

In addition to mind traffic, the night season can be disrupted through nightmares and bad dreams. It is important to remember that not all dreams are from the enemy. There are three basic sources for our dreams: God, the demonic, and our own soul. While it is not the topic of this book to examine dreams in full, it is essential to remember that God uses dreams as one of the ways He chooses to communicate with His people (i.e., Joseph's and Daniel's dreams in Scripture). As a result, the enemy's efforts to disrupt the night season through nightmares and bad dreams can be seen as an effort to destroy the willingness of an individual to listen to this type of communication from God. God dreams go beyond what might simply be called "good" dreams and enter the realm of spiritual communication. Dreams that come from our own soul can add to the confusion that makes it difficult to differentiate what needs to be taken seriously and what needs to be dismissed. Soul dreams can result from our mind's concentration on what we want or desire, from drugs (legal, illegal, prescription, and non-prescription) and alcohol, and even from foods we eat. While it is possible for such dreams to have some spiritual significance, most frequently they do not. What might be considered good and/or bad dreams can both come from the soul. Frequently referred to as nightmares, dreams inspired by demonic oppression can be a major element of the enemy's plan to disrupt the night season, and as a result, they should be dealt with on a spiritual level.

People attempt to deal with these issues of the night in many different ways. Some individuals turn to counselors to seek assistance in restoring peaceful sleep, and others turn to medications. When applied to a spiritual issue, these solutions typically only provide temporary relief. Issues of the night season that result from demonic oppression must be dealt with on a spiritual basis. The heart of dealing with the matter is found in confession, repentance, and forgiveness as they are explained earlier in this book.

For more immediate relief and when others are not available to assist with the process of walking into freedom from such oppression, it can be quite helpful to take action that helps change the atmosphere around you. The best way to do this is to play an audio version of the Bible through the night. The volume level should be turned down to a level just below readily perceptible, to a point where the individual can listen and follow along with the Scripture being read if they concentrate to do so. This keeps the volume level just low enough that the sound itself does not interfere with sleep and just loud enough to be discerned as the spirit-man listens. In particular, it can be very helpful to listen to passages taken from the Psalms and to avoid passages from books such as Revelation. This technique helps to calm the mind, soothe the spirit, frustrate the demonic, and it allows peace to return until the situation can be dealt with in a more direct fashion.

War Stories

Catchers

While the need to deal with the demonic is much the same around the world, the common practices and methods of ministry can be quite diverse. In Africa, a typical church service will include a ministry team well prepared to enter the midst of the congregation and physically carry from the room those in whom a demon is manifesting through screams or flailing of the body upon the floor. In South America, the deliverance minister often uses a mixture of traditional Catholic exorcism practices, mixed with more "charismatic" techniques such as those mentioned here. In traveling around the world, we have noticed something important: ministry teams everywhere often function on high levels of ritual, moderate levels of power, and limited levels of authority. If we are to see true success in deliverance, it is essential that we learn to increase the level of authority, while decreasing the level of ritual involved in our ministry.

While observing a deliverance team in Africa, Michael once served as a "catcher" for the team. In typical Pentecostal or charismatic churches the term "catcher" would refer to the individual whose job it was to "catch" a person who falls (usually backward) under the power of God. The term took on new meaning in Africa where Michael was expected to "catch" any of the individuals who decided to make a break for it through the room's only exit. Because this practice was so entrenched culturally, it typically took several strong men to guard the door when various individuals rushed it in an effort to depart the area. While this practice of forcing an individual to remain confined until the demon was dealt with would meet with much disapproval in the United States, it is frequently the order of the day in Africa. After standing with the team at the door for some time and wandering throughout the room to both assist and observe, a curious fact became apparent. When Michael was at the door exercising the God-given authority that was present in his life, individuals would start toward the door and generally stop and turn around about five feet or so before they reached it. On the other hand, when the "nervous" catchers were at the door, hoping not to let someone slip through their grasp, there were frequent occasions when wrestling matches ensued to keep the individuals from "escaping." While this observation did not hold completely true for every situation, it clearly indicates that it can be easy to slip into a method of ministry that is functioning out of our own strength (catching people at the door) and not even realize that authority is available to deal with the issue far more effectively. It is important to remember that the demonic can impart supernatural strength such as it did with the Gadarene demoniac,[94] and thus operating in our own strength can at times be both difficult and dangerous.

Hold That Bible

On a visit to India, Michael and a team had the opportunity to minister to a young lady who had been deeply troubled by the demonic for some time. The events that took place provide a wonderful illustration of why it is not only of spiritual significance, but also of practical importance to distinguish between dealing with the demonic entity and the individual receiving ministry. As might be expected, there was some difficulty associated with the fact that Michael does not speak Hindi, and the young lady needed an interpreter to understand English. The pastor knew that the team was coming, but had not told the congregation because in some parts of India a relationship with American "preachers" is looked down upon as the people sometimes believe that their leaders become puppets to American money. In the two weeks before the team's arrival, it became apparent that the demonic *was* aware that they were coming, in that it was stirred up significantly in this young lady—to the point that she attempted suicide at least twice before they arrived.

While the young lady herself had been a Christian for some time, her mother was a recent convert, and the pastor was unsure as to how she would react to a group of Americans ministering deliverance to her daughter. As it turned out, the Holy Spirit had revealed to the mother that people were coming from far away to help her daughter get free, and when the team arrived the mother was both happy and very cooperative. As ministry began, the young lady became somewhat violent and would shout in Hindi and slap at the people around her. She kept repeating a Hindi word and at one point Michael finally asked what the word meant. To everyone's surprise, an immediate response came from the lips of the young lady receiving ministry. She answered in perfect English and explained what the word meant, then almost as quickly and still in perfect English said, "Why did you tell him that?" She then refused to speak at all. The two demonic beings assaulting her understood and spoke English and were conversing with each other.

Deliverance was going slowly, and one of the difficulties seemed to be in getting the young lady to understand that she had to exercise her own authority over the demonic, as well. Through the interpreter, the team attempted to explain this concept and have her speak out loud that she wanted the demon to leave, but something was either lost in translation or she simply could not exercise sufficient control over her own voice to make the declaration. Michael had placed his Bible in her lap several times and each time she had slapped it away. So instead of Michael continuing to try to get her to speak, the Lord impressed upon him to have her hold the Bible as a declaration of her will that she desired to be free. Looking into her eyes, but speaking through an interpreter, he explained what he wanted her to do and then handed her the Bible. You might expect that she took hold of it and immediately received her freedom, but that was not the case. Instead, she took the Bible and threw it across the room. After hearing what the team wanted her to do several more times and understanding what was being said (note the importance of distinguishing between speaking to the demon and speaking to the individual that is illustrated here), she was able with great struggle to hold the Bible in her hands as a sign that she wanted the demon to leave. A short time after this "declaration," the battle that had raged for several hours ended with her being set free. By ensuring that the individual understood and cooperated in receiving her deliverance and that the demonic entity could not interfere with their ability to express that desire, freedom became a much easier goal to obtain for her.

Over the Shoulder

When you are willing to help people obtain their freedom from the demonic, it is usually not necessary to go out and look for people who need freedom; instead, they are often led across your path. One night during an evening prayer service at their church, Michael and Bill were faced with a young man who obviously needed help. He entered the building and "interrupted" the service looking for another minister. After hearing that the person was not available, the young man became very agitated. When asked what he needed, he boldly said, "Deliverance!" Michael explained that those present for the church service would be glad to pray for him and minister to him, but he was insistent that only the minister he had asked for could help. He became outraged when Michael would not provide the home telephone number of the one he was looking for and insisted that he was going to go through the building and look for him. Since the young man was somewhat small in stature, no one anticipated any particular danger and so, turning the service over to someone else, Michael began to escort the man to a room while explaining that they would be glad to pray for him. Once again the young man became outraged and Michael pointed at him and said, "In the name of Jesus..." In the blink of an eye, the young man grabbed Michael's arm and threw him over his shoulder, into the air, and across the room, then jumped onto him on the floor and began hitting him.

First, it should be pointed out that Michael was not hurt at all. This is a clear application of Luke 10:19, that when we know who we are in Christ and understand our power and authority over the enemy, nothing shall hurt us. The second point that can be learned from this experience is that our first reactions (no matter how much experience we have in the realm of deliverance ministry) will often be to act in our own strength. If this happens, it is important to return to a spiritual perspective as quickly as possible. When Michael was thrown to the floor, not only did he attempt to fight back and free himself, but Bill and other leaders came to his aid in attempting to pull the young man off of him, through their own physical strength. After a few moments of struggle, Michael realized the enemy's tactic and simply touched the young man on the shoulder and gently declared, "Peace, in the name of Jesus." The young man went immediately limp and lay down flat on the floor. Getting him up and into a chair, the spontaneous deliverance team was able to minister to him and see him freed from a spirit of violence and other oppressive demonic entities.

Worship Warfare

As has already been suggested, worship can be an excellent weapon in our warfare against the demonic. This can be both as an intentional decision to worship in the face of an onslaught of the enemy, or warfare can be initiated simply as a byproduct of the worship environment. On frequent occasions, those involved in deliverance will notice that the demonic world is stirred up during times of worship. In Africa, worship is often used as a tool of spiritual warfare and engaged in with the specific intention of provoking the demonic to reveal itself. In such worship settings, African deliverance teams often have two or three men and women prepared to enter the room and literally carry out anyone whose physical responses are overwhelmed by a demonic manifestation. They are often taken to another room where a ministry team can take time with them to help them get free from the demonic.

Worship is equally powerful in stirring up the demonic. On one occasion during a local church service where Michael was preaching, a woman from a very traditional church background approached his wife Elisa at the front of the sanctuary. She expressed concern that something was going on in her body physically and that she felt like she just needed to scream. Elisa kindly escorted her to the rear of the sanctuary and sent word for Bill to come and help deal with the issue. After a short prayer and a brief explanation of the possible need for deliverance, the woman insisted that she still needed to scream. Bill and Elisa told her to go ahead, and her scream was quite clear even over the sounds of ongoing worship. After a bit more ministry, the woman indicated that she still felt as though she needed to scream and did so once again—long and loudly. At this point, with joy clearly showing upon her face, she turned to Bill and Elisa and said, "I feel so different, like I am free." Most of the congregation was so involved in worship that they never even noticed what was taking place. Deliverance had been surprisingly unobtrusive and simple. She left the service free as much a result of the warfare that had taken place through the worship, as from the prayers and ministry of the team.

Biblically, worship can clearly be identified as a part of both active warfare and a catalyst for peace. Jehoshaphat's obedience to the Lord's instruction that he send worshipers before his army against overwhelming odds in 2 Chronicles 20 is an illustration of worship literally changing the course of a physical battle. In 1 Samuel 16, we find David using worship as a means of imparting peace to a situation in which King Saul fell under the tormenting influence of a demonic entity. In one case the enemy was stirred into such a frenzy that they began to turn upon themselves (much like the use of worship in Africa to provoke a demonic entity to reveal itself), and in the other, worship brought relief from torment by calming the demonic manifestation in Saul's life.

FINAL THOUGHTS:
WHAT DO I DO NOW?

Three categories of people have likely read this book:

1. Those who are intrigued by what they've read and will ponder it in their hearts until the opportune time.

2. Those who are called to deliverance ministry and are ready to jump in with both feet.

3. Those who never want to hear the word *deliverance* again.

The Holy Spirit will direct the steps of the first two groups and bring those in need across their path. For members of the final group, though the Holy Spirit may test their willingness to act on His behalf, He will never force them to violate their will. No one has to use the information contained in these pages; undoubtedly, though, God has directed you to this book for a reason. If you choose not to apply what you've read here, you and those you could have helped will miss out. These principles of deliverance will mature those who pursue them. New understanding will come with each opportunity to touch the life of another.

Now that you have a clearer understanding of who your enemy is and what he does, you should be able to walk much more consistently in 2 Timothy 1:7, which states that God has not given us a spirit of fear, but of power, love, and a sound mind. True, we face a powerful, cunning adversary, but we need not fear him because God has given us authority over his power. In fact, knowing who he is and what he does should give us more confidence to oppose him. Even if the enemy were to exert every ounce of his strength, our power is greater. The love of God resident in our heart carries more authority, and the soundness of our mind enables us to confront him boldly. As a Christian, if we can fully apprehend this spiritual truth, then we need not fear the demonic having any impact in our life.

Deliverance ministry does not begin or end with commanding demons to go. In fact, preparation for ministry is perhaps more important than the actual ministry itself. The time spent preparing our heart is when the Lord fills us with the power we need to minister. Recognize that our adversary wants to distract us with the flaws that surface in those in need. Preparation and ministry are essential, but follow-up is also imperative. If we've securely laid the foundation from the beginning of the process, follow-up should be relatively simple. Usually, when someone begins to walk in true freedom, accompanying it is an innate desire to remain free.

Ultimately, every soldier must still follow the rules of engagement to remain covered by the Lord's protection. We must recognize that while God has given us tremendous freedom to act, function, and minister in His name, we must honor the boundaries He has established if we are to be effective and safe. The boundaries for ministry identified in this book should not be viewed as restrictions, but as guidelines that help us remain covered by the Lord's protection. God's Word has layers of meaning, from the overtly practical to the deeply spiritual, and the following story, while somewhat humorous after the fact, illustrates this point.

In the early days of his deliverance ministry, Bill did everything he perceived a "good" Christian minister should do. Each time he ministered, he would follow the same pattern. He dressed nicely in slacks, dress shirt, and tie. He would greet the person seeking help and then begin ministry by bowing his head, closing his eyes, and praying. One day, while he was ministering in this manner, the young woman for whom he was praying began acting under demonic influence and calmly reached forward (unbeknownst to Bill, whose eyes were closed) and grabbed him by the tie, wrenching downward. Bill eventually freed himself from her grasp, but he learned a valuable lesson clearly stated in Scripture.

> "Watch *therefore, and pray always that you may be counted worthy to escape all these things that will come to pass, and to stand before the Son of Man.*"
> —*Luke 21:36* NKJV *(emphasis added)*

This passage has taken on new meaning to Bill ever since. When ministering deliverance, never close your eyes, but watch while you pray so that you may escape the enemy's plans. If you are uncomfortable praying with your eyes open, you may wish to forego the necktie!

Finally, the Holy Spirit is the power that does the ministry, not us. If you truly understand this, you won't be distracted by arguments over whether or not a person has to speak in tongues, etc. You will be able to recognize the Holy Spirit's power, and you will find it much easier to handle the situations the Lord allows to come before you.

What you have freely received needs to be freely given. As a believer, you have every right, and the responsibility, to help others understand what it takes to achieve and maintain freedom. Jesus never freed someone from a demonic strongman before he or she was ready. An important part of the deliverance process is understanding how to close—and also being willing to close—the door that was opened by our own sin or the sin of another. So, remember to teach and lead people to confess, repent, and forgive before utilizing the authority, power, and weapons at our disposal. God is not in the business of violating the free will of any individual, so for our weapons to be effective, those we minister to must *want* to be free. The desire for freedom is directly proportional to the willingness to prepare through confession, repentance, and forgiveness.

***

I (Michael) wrote this final chapter while sitting along the Gulf Coast of Alabama, listening to the sounds of the surf coming in and watching the waves toss themselves against the beach. An osprey (a large fish-eating bird resembling an eagle) flew past my window and back and forth along the beach. In that moment, the Lord spoke to me about how different individuals approach deliverance ministry. Some are like the osprey floating on the winds and searching for the right moment to plunge after its prey.

The Lord directed my attention to the osprey as an example of how a deliverance minister operates in the Spirit. He pointed out how the osprey soars, using its keen eyesight to search for fish just below the water's surface. Sometimes it dives toward the ocean, only to pull up and away at the last moment, without piercing the water. But then, suddenly, with clear determination, it plunges and almost disappears into the sea. Although struggling, it soon emerges from the water, and with determined effort, lifts once again into the air, carrying its catch home to its nest.

The Lord told me He wanted His people to approach deliverance ministry in the same way this bird carries out its appointed task. To properly function in this ministry, we must be willing to float upon the wind of the Spirit and use the piercing eyes of our heart to delve below the surface of the lives that come our way. There will be times when we see people and know they are ready to be pulled from the enemy's clutches, yet when we approach them, they dart away into the depths and slip too far beneath the surface to be reached. But as we continue following the Spirit and watching for opportunities the Lord will supply, the time will come when that determined plunge will bring freedom to the one the Lord has shown us. While it will no doubt require some degree of struggle, and at times the weight of this responsibility may seem greater than we can bear, perseverance will bring results. We will have the opportunity to lead people out of the darkness and home to the enveloping love of God.

About the Authors

MICHAEL FRENCH, B.A., M.P.A., J.D.
After practicing law for ten years, Michael received his call into the ministry. Over the past twenty-seven years, he has passionately ministered all around the globe. Michael is the founder of Cahaba Equipping Center, a ministry devoted to training and equipping leaders around the world. Michael is also the co-founder and executive director of Patria Ministries, an international association of churches and ministries headquartered in Birmingham, Alabama. Michael and his wife Elisa live in Leeds, Alabama, with their four sons, Joshua, Caleb, Jacob, and Noah.

BILL FRENCH

Bill is the founder of Advocate Ministries and has been involved in ministry for more than thirty-five years (at the time of this book), with much of that time devoted to counseling those who have been involved in the occult. Bill has been married to his wife, Joyce, for sixty-two years. He has four children (Barry, Renee, Michael, and Leslee), eleven grandchildren, and nine great-grandchildren. While his work as a counselor has ended, at his current age of eighty-nine, he continues to travel and speak on issues related to overcoming the demonic and (as Bill likes to say) on the "whole counsel of the Word of God."

Authors' Acknowledgments

We wish to acknowledge the hundreds of people who have trusted this ministry with their spiritual (and sometimes physical) lives as they endeavored to overcome the demonic realm.

It is also important to recognize the commitment of the staff of Advocate Ministries, The Bridge Birmingham (formerly

Cahaba Christian Fellowship). The former and current staff from both these ministries have carried our burdens as the pages of this book were written and lived out.

We also recognize the Freedom Night Ministry Team. The individuals who have worked side by side with Bill over the years are too numerous to count. These men and women stand with us and beside us in all we do, never flinching in the face of spiritual warfare. Learning and implementing the principles described here have subjected us and those around us to many attacks of the enemy, but he has never been victorious.

We would also like to thank John Paul Jackson, Greg and Patty Mapes, and the entire team at Streams Ministries. Without your help, this project might never have gone beyond Michael's computer screen.

Jennifer Minigh and the team at Shade Tree Publishing also deserve acknowledgement for inspiring and drawing out more from us in this revised and updated edition.

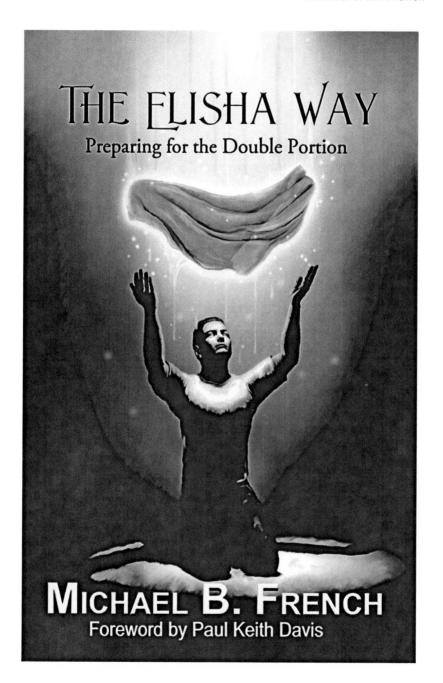

THE ELISHA WAY

Preparing for the Double Portion

MICHAEL B. FRENCH

Foreword by Paul Keith Davis

Remedy: Freedom Through Deliverance

References and Scriptures

1 Philippians 2:25; 2 Timothy 2:3–4

2 John 10:10

3 Isaiah 14:16–17 NKJV

4 Revelation 12:4–9

5 Luke 10:19

6 2 Corinthians 11:14

7 Genesis 2:17

8 2 Peter 3:8 NKJV

9 Luke 22:31

10 Luke 22:32

11 Job 1:21 NKJV

12 Job 2:3–6

13 Zechariah 3

14 Deuteronomy 32:17; Psalm 106:37

15 Leviticus 17:7; 2 Chronicles 11:15

16 Luke 11:20

17 John R. Kohlenberger III and James A. Swanson, eds., *The Strongest Strong's Exhaustive Concordance of the Bible* (Grand Rapids: Zondervan, 2001).

18 John 10:10

19 *Biblesoft's New Exhaustive Strong's Numbers and Concordance with Expanded Greek-Hebrew Dictionary* (Biblesoft and International Bible Translators, Inc., 1994).

20 Jewish tradition held that a parent was responsible for a child's keeping of the law until he or she reached adulthood. For a boy, this happened at the age of thirteen, and the celebration of this rite of passage is called *bar mitzvah* ("son of the commandment"), acknowledging that the child has now become accountable to keep the commandments himself. Otherwise, if the parent were still responsible for the child's keeping the law, one could conclude that the parent's faith would suffice to set the child free.

21 Romans 7:18

22 Romans 13:14

23 Romans 12:2

24 Romans 8:7

25 Philippians 2:5

26 Galatians 3:7 NKJV

27 1 Samuel 18:10–11

28 Matthew 10:7–8

29 John 8:44

30 Ephesians 4:7 NKJV

31 Ephesians 4:12–13

32 Philippians 2:10

33 Revelation 12:9

34 *Biblesoft's New Exhaustive Strong's Numbers and Concordance with Expanded Greek-Hebrew Dictionary.* (Copyright © 1994, 2003, 2006 Biblesoft, Inc. and International Bible Translators, Inc.).

35 Acts 8:18 NKJV

36 *American Heritage Dictionary of the English Language* (Boston: Houghton Mifflin Company, 2000).

37 Mark 11:23

38 *Thayer's Greek Lexicon*, Electronic Database. (Copyright © 2000, 2003, 2006 by Biblesoft, Inc.).

39 John 5:19

40 John 14:15
41 Romans 12:11 NKJV
42 Ephesians 6:13
43 Ephesians 4:13
44 Acts 16:18
45 Matthew 17:21
46 Psalm 69:5
47 2 Thessalonians 3:13
48 Romans 8:13–14
49 John 10:10
50 Matthew 4:4, 7, 10
51 Romans 8:5–7
52 Romans 12:2
53 1 Corinthians 14:14
54 Jude 1:20
55 2 Chronicles 20
56 Isaiah 60:18
57 1 John 2:9–11
58 Mark 9:18–19
59 Matthew 6:25–30
60 Matthew 9:22; Mark 10:52
61 Mark 4:24; Luke 8:18
62 Romans 10:17
63 John 17:17
64 John 8:32 NKJV
65 Romans 6:6–11
66 Romans 7:19
67 James 4:7
68 1 Peter 5:8–9
69 James 4:4
70 1 Peter 5:5–6
71 Matthew 6:13
72 Matthew 6:11
73 1 Corinthians 9:27
74 Matthew 7:14
75 Matthew 6:16–18
76 1 Timothy 6:12
77 Genesis 3
78 Matthew 4
79 Luke 8:26–33
80 Mark 6:12–13
81 James 2:19
82 Luke 10:19
83 Genesis 1:26
84 Matthew 28:18 NKJV
85 John 14:12
86 Matthew 5:48
87 Mark 7:14–23
88 James 1:14–15; Galatians 5:19–21
89 Romans 6:15–16
90 John 14:30 NKJV
91 Matthew 5:21–22 NKJV
92 Hebrews 13:2
93 1 Corinthians 12:12
94 Mark 5:1–5

CPSIA information can be obtained at www.ICGtesting.com
Printed in the USA
BVOW05s1019020714

358018BV00003B/125/P